Acquiring Interpersonal Skills

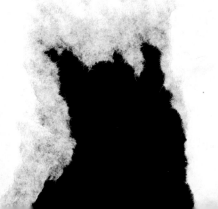

Acquiring Interpersonal Skills

A HANDBOOK OF EXPERIENTIAL LEARNING FOR HEALTH PROFESSIONALS

Second Edition

Philip Burnard

University of Wales College of Medicine, Cardiff

Stanley Thornes (Publishers) Ltd

First edition published in 1989 by Chapman & Hall (as *Teaching Interpersonal Skills: A Handbook of Experiential Learning for Health Professionals*)
Second edition published by Chapman & Hall 1996

Reprinted in 1999 by:
Stanley Thornes (Publishers) Ltd
Ellenborough House
Wellington Street
Cheltenham
Glos.
GL50 1YW
United Kingdom

99 00 01 02 03 / 10 9 8 7 6 5 4 3 2 1

A catalogue record for this book is available from the British Library

ISBN 0–7487–4589–0

Typeset by Saxon Graphics Ltd, Derby
Printed and bound in Great Britain by Athenaeum Press Ltd, Gateshead, Tyne & Wear

As always, for Sally, Aaron and Rebecca

Contents

Preface

Health care, in Britain at least, has changed dramatically since the publication of the first edition of this book. We have seen the way in which health care is funded change considerably. We have seen a call for greater accountability by individuals within the health services, cuts to publicly funded health care, the closure of hospitals and the development of the private sector. There has also been a dramatic shift in the training of all health care workers towards the higher education sector. New universities have opened up new health care departments. Many health care professionals who would, only fairly recently, have trained in local colleges now undertake university courses and graduate with degrees in their respective professions. Cross-discipline teaching is also a feature of these changes. It can be anticipated that within the next ten years medical students, nursing students and various therapy students will all be taught together.

With the increasing emphasis on quality assurance and on the evaluation of care has come an even greater need for all health professionals to consider their own interpersonal skills. Such skills range from the very simple – client/staff introductions – to the more elaborate, such as psychotherapy and counselling. To reflect some of these changes and, I hope, to enhance the value of this book, I have introduced the following features into this new edition:

- more critical debate about the issues involved;
- more examples and activities;
- more reporting of other people's work;
- reports of research into interpersonal skills and interpersonal skills training;
- details of how to run courses with larger numbers of students;
- details of training larger numbers of people in 'presentation skills'.

In these, and many other respects, I am indebted to people in the field who have commented on the first edition and offered suggestions for the second. I have tried to incorporate as many of those ideas as possible into this edition.

The climate in education continues to change. In some ways, we have seen something of a shift back to 'teacher-centred' methods in colleges and universities. This book continues to recommend that the only real way of developing interpersonal skills is to practise them. No amount of lecturing or reading can ever replace experience in this field. Therefore, although I address the question of lecturers and seminars, I remain convinced that experiential learning methods – however they are defined – remain the best way of learning about how to relate to others in health care settings.

This book is aimed at anyone in the health professions who is concerned about enhancing interpersonal competence, either their own or other people's. It also tells you how to achieve this aim. The chapters that follow offer both theories and also guidance in practice. The book contains many practical illustrations of 'how-to-do-it' and a longer, illustrative package that tries to convey the running of a typical interpersonal skills workshop.

The first chapter offers a fairly detailed analysis of the concept of experiential learning: the notion of learning through personal experience and the notion on which this book is based. The second chapter offers the reader some practical examples of the wide range of experiential learning methods available to her and notes on how to use them in interpersonal skills training. The third chapter discusses examples of interpersonal skills for use in the health professions and argues that a thorough grounding in counselling skills can enable the health professional to develop other interpersonal skills.

The next few chapters offer details of how to organize, set up and run interpersonal skills training workshops and groups, with examples from practice. The penultimate chapter supplies a range of clearly laid out exercises for use in such workshops and groups. The final chapter – a new one – offers a rather different approach to skills training based on the changing face of health care. It argues for bringing all health care professionals up to a basic level of attainment in what I have called 'presentation skills'. The chapter offers a model for thinking about training health care workers in larger groups and in relatively short periods of time. In many ways, it is an 'experimental' chapter and the full implications of it have yet to be fully worked out. I have consulted a number of large business organizations for ideas about this chapter and I am grateful to them for their help. I believe that we have to look, constantly, at new ways of doing things in what is always a changing health care climate. Some of the more obviously 'humanistic' ways of training people are, perhaps, less appropriate today. That is not to suggest in any way that we must lose sight of our own or our clients' 'humanity' but simply to note that time and ideas move on.

A conclusion summarizes many of the main points of the book and offers some practical elaboration of them. It can be used as a checklist when thinking about organizing interpersonal skills training sessions. The book closes with a detailed bibliography of further and recommended reading. The reader should find it useful as a source of material for further study and practice.

I learned to use the approaches described in this book by using them in training a variety of health care professionals in counselling, experiential learning, stress management, group facilitation, managing change, self-awareness and curriculum development over a period of more than 15 years. In writing this volume, I hope that a variety of health professionals, from nurses to social workers and from occupational therapists to GPs will find the approach easier than they thought and will enjoy the experience of experimenting with the exercises and activities contained in it.

While the book is primarily written for trainers and lecturers in the health professions, it may also be useful to the clinical practitioner who wishes to develop expertise in helping patients and clients to enhance their interpersonal skills. In the fields of social work, health visiting and psychiatric nursing, for example, there are numerous occasions on which the development of conversational and social skills can help improve personal performance and self-awareness. The awareness of basic counselling and group skills can also do much to improve the quality of communication between people in families and organizations.

Like many other writers, I still have difficulties in solving the problem of how to write in non-sexist language. I considered using 'they' as both singular and plural but that seemed clumsy. Alternate chapters of 'he' and 'she' seemed equally awkward. I have settled for using 'she' to described the facilitator of interpersonal learning groups. Please read 'he' when this is appropriate.

Philip Burnard,
Caerphilly,
Mid Glamorgan,
Wales.

Whoever you are holding me now in hand,
Without one thing all will be useless,
I give you fair warning before you attempt me further
I am not what you supposed, but far different.

(Walt Whitman, 1860)

Learning from life: experiential learning

We all learn from experience. That is not to say that we learn everything from experience nor to suggest that we always learn from experience. A moment's reflection will reveal how often that is not the case. I am constantly horrified by how often I do the same things and make the same mistakes ... and haven't learned much in the process. Or, as Kurt Vonnegut, the American humourist, put it:

> That is my principle objection to life, I think: it is too easy, when alive, to make perfectly horrible mistakes (Vonnegut, 1983).

On the other hand, I am equally surprised how often I have learned the really important things in my life, not from books, nor from being told things by other people, but from having had something happen to me that I have found interesting or important. This is experiential learning. So, of course, is learning from some of our mistakes and from some of the mistakes of others. This latter form of learning is sometimes known as **vicarious** learning. We don't have to experience everything ourselves, in order to learn. It is quite possible to watch someone fall of a ladder, for example, and to realize that the experience is not for us and, also, to learn quite a bit about the placement and stability of ladders. So, too, do we learn vicariously in the interpersonal world. We see people interacting with each other and, from a very early age, appreciate the differences between someone who is polite, friendly and interpersonally skilled and someone who is not. We then adopt (either consciously or otherwise) those behaviours and skills that we deem to be appropriate and effective. And this process continues, to a greater and lesser extent, throughout life. We are constantly 'fine tuning' our behaviour or trying out new ways of interacting. It seems unlikely that this is a linear process. I doubt that we change constantly and at the same sort of rate throughout our lives. It seems more likely that there are 'bursts' of learning at different points in our lives with smaller changes taking place in between.

In a sense, of course, almost **all** learning is experiential: the very fact of learning something at all is an experience. However, the term has come to be used in certain ways to denote a style of learning from personal, 'hands-on' experience. As we shall see, it has been variously defined and by different sorts of commentators. What binds all of the definitions and writers together is the importance placed on how I – as a living human being – can benefit from taking note of what happens to me and how I can take what I learn from everyday situations to new situations in the future. None of us is simply a learning machine. We do not just take in information and facts, process them and file them away. We are in constant, day-to-day interaction with our surroundings and, in particular, with other people, like us. All of this interaction helps us to think and feel about ourselves and about others and causes us to respond.

All of the health care professions are very much **responding** professions. This reflective, thoughtful process is also an important part of experiential learning. For experiential learning, at its best (and probably also at its most basic) takes us beyond book theories to personal responses. For I suspect that most of us do not live our lives out of books. Even if we teach out of them, we often have cause to question them. If we are academics and teachers, we often have a 'private' and 'real' side that works up alongside the more 'academic' side. And those two are sometimes congruent and sometimes incongruent. I have yet to meet, for example, a psychologist who followed all of the precepts of psychology. Life, I suspect, is lived at a more basic and more immediate level. Learning to notice how we live our lives is also part of that broad category of ideas and theories called experiential learning.

This, immediately, raises a problem – for this is a book about experiential learning and about relationships. It would seem that, at one level, I am contradicting myself. For if we do not learn about relationships from books, then why write one on the topic? I would answer, in defence, that this book, like so many others, can only offer a structure or a framework for thinking about the topic. There are no hard and fast rules about what constitutes a 'good' or 'appropriate' interpersonal skill. For one thing, interpersonal skills are very much **contextual** and dependent upon a huge range of variables including the people involved, the environment, the relationships between them, the time and so on. Nor are there particular rules about teaching those skills (the one point must follow the other). It has been my experience, though, that many people are worried about approaching the subject at all because of not knowing where to start. This book, then, offers a sounding board for your own ideas.

It also needs to be said at the outset that the field of interpersonal skills is awash with theory. There are theories about how counselling 'works' and how best to handle people who are distressed. There are theories about how to train others in the social skills that they are seen to lack. There are even theories about how the mind works, how dreams do or do not work and so on. The point, perhaps, is to remember that they **are** theories and not to let them 'slide' into becoming facts – to reify them. Part of the process of developing experiential learning methods is also a process of becoming critical. Everything, I suggest, can be usefully held up for criticism and this must include the range of theories that have been developed in this chapter, in other chapters and in other books. For we still know remarkably little about how people 'work'. If we want to progress as health professionals in the 'caring' side of those professions, then our task is to move slowly and to generalize only with extreme caution. If we do not, we stand to tread on the thoughts and feelings of the people for whom we care. By forcing our theories on them – however benign those theories might be – we stand to misuse the power we have as professionals. We need to bear this in mind, too, as teachers of student health professionals. In sharing our experiences with students, we need to tread lightly. For if we do not, we stand to offer not facilitation but indoctrination.

On the other hand, this, too, raises problems. We cannot be atheoretical. Like it or not, we all have beliefs and theories about why people are as they are. These may be fully worked out or they may be at the level of 'I have met a lot of people in my time and experience has taught me...' level. We may also have conflicting and contradictory theories about people's behaviour. We may even have a 'two-tier' theory system: a set of theories about people that we expound in public and another 'personal' set of theories. This is sometimes the case with people who teach in the behavioural and interpersonal domain. The counselling skills trainer may, for example, teach a 'client-centred' approach to working with other people, while being fairly directive or even bossy in his or her personal life. We probably have to accept that, as human beings, we are contrary, often inconsistent and subject to various paradoxes. All of this can make interpersonal skills training more, rather than less, interesting.

The ideas in this chapter, then, and in this book, are provisional. They do not represent the view of how interpersonal skills might be encouraged but raise pointers for thinking about teaching interpersonal skills. The real teaching and learning come from the personal interactions between teachers and their students and from the relationships that develop between students and their clients. The odd request, then, is to read this book in a critical spirit. To question and challenge the ideas in it and to take them up only with some caution.

The chapter begins with a discussion of some definitions of experiential learning and noting how the concept of experiential learning may be applied in health care settings. it then goes on to define three types of knowledge and offers a revised definition of experiential learning in terms of this theory. An historical view of the topic is then given and, finally, the particular characteristics of experiential learning are identified and enumerated.

ACQUIRING INTERPERSONAL SKILLS IN THE HEALTH PROFESSIONS: NUMBER 1

Awareness

Awareness is the simple process of noticing what is going on around you. Most of the time, we are caught up with our own thoughts and feelings and fail to observe the world surrounding us. The conscious practice of 'staying awake' and noticing what we and others do can help us to improve our interpersonal skills. We cannot change unless we choose to. We cannot change unless we notice what we do.

The process of 'noticing' is essential to acquiring interpersonal skills. This is not an activity to carry out 'part time' but a skill to develop over time. It might be argued that the truly skilled person is one who is 'noticing' all of the time.

EXPERIENTIAL LEARNING DEFINED

Experiential learning is learning through doing. It is also more than that. It is learning through reflecting on the doing. In all aspects of our actions, we have at least two choices: just to act or to notice how we act. It is only through noticing what it is that we do that we can hope to learn about ourselves and our behaviour. To 'just act' is to act blindly, unawarely. This is what happens when we do not learn from experience. In a sense, it is as simple as that: if we are to learn from what we do, we must notice what we do and reflect on it. To notice what we do is to allow ourselves to evaluate action and to choose the next piece of behaviour. This is living in a more precise way. Now clearly we cannot notice our behaviour and actions all the time. But in terms of the relationships we have with our clients, we owe it to them to notice our behaviour more frequently than we may be doing at present. To do this noticing is to engage in what Heron (1973) calls 'conscious use of the self': using behaviour and the self in a conscious, therapeutic manner. To make conscious use of the self during interpersonal relationships is to enhance the likeliness of our relationships being therapeutic.

On the other hand, of course, there is an inherent contradiction running through this idea. For if we are to make conscious use of the self, to what are we referring as the doer of this action? If the 'self' is the actor, then it cannot also be the observer of the action. This is a contradiction that we will meet later in the book in the section on self-awareness and it is not an easy one to resolve.

There is a second meaning of the term experiential learning. We all learn through experience, whether directly, through taking action, through being involved in a situation or by observing others. In this sense, every situation is an experiential learning situation. To describe experiential learning in such broad terms would be rather fruitless, however, it would make the concept so huge as to render it unmanageable. To make things a little clearer, we may identify four aspects of experiential learning:

1. personal experience;
2. reflection on that experience;
3. the transformation of knowledge and meaning as a result of that reflection;
4. application of that transformed knowledge into practical action.

EXAMPLES OF EXPERIENTIAL LEARNING IN THE HEALTH CARE FIELD

All health professionals learn through reflecting on their practice. Experiential learning does not occur, as we have noted, when we do not reflect on our practice. The issue of reflection is a crucial one. In order to learn, we must first notice or, as Ouspensky (1988) put it, we must learn to remember ourselves. Ouspensky argues that for much of our lives we are only half conscious or we are working on 'automatic pilot'. When we do this, we no longer register what is happening to us. Indeed, Ouspensky argues that if we do not remember ourselves and notice what is happening to us, we will not commit to memory the events that are taking place within and around us. Instead, we must learn to cultivate an increasing awareness of our senses and of our changing thoughts, feelings and actions. Examples of how this reflective ability can help us to learn in the health professions are as follows. A reflective ability can help us in:

- learning through talking to clients;
- working in the field;
- reflecting on past clinical experiences;
- comparing notes with other health care professionals;
- noticing personal thoughts, feelings and emotions;
- exploring feelings in small groups;
- attendance at experiential learning workshops;
- learning counselling and group therapy by working with clients;
- keeping journals and diaries;
- receiving positive and negative feedback from colleagues and peers;
- comparing past and present situations;
- using relaxation and meditational activities;
- consciously managing time;
- using problem-solving devices and strategies;
- entering into personal therapy/counselling;
- consciously trying new coping strategies;
- learning by 'sitting with Nellie': learning on the job;
- trial and error learning;

- learning by experimentation;
- reading about, then trying out, new ideas;
- consciously changing role;
- practising new interpersonal skills;
- learning group facilitation by running groups.

ACQUIRING INTERPERSONAL SKILLS IN THE HEALTH PROFESSIONS: NUMBER 2

Self-description

Try writing out a description of yourself in the third person. That is to say, start the description as follows: 'John Smith is an interesting person who ...'. The process of doing this can add insight into how we perceive ourselves and how we think others perceive us. This activity can also be used as a group exercise. Each person writes out their own self-description and then shares it with the rest of the group. Each person may also ask for feedback on their particular description.

EXPERIENTIAL LEARNING AS THE DEVELOPMENT OF EXPERIENTIAL KNOWLEDGE

Another approach to appreciating the notion of experiential learning comes through discussion of types of knowledge. Three types of knowledge that go to make up an individual may be described: propositional knowledge, practical knowledge and experiential knowledge (Heron, 1981). While each of these types is different, each is interrelated with the other. Thus, while propositional knowledge may be considered as qualitatively different to, say, practical knowledge, it is possible and probably better, to use propositional knowledge in the application of practical knowledge. The discussion, here, started from Heron's position but also moves away from it in various ways.

Propositional knowledge

Propositional knowledge is that which is contained in theories or models. Literally, propositional knowledge is made up of statements and propositions. It may be described as 'textbook' knowledge and is synonymous with Ryle's (1949) concept of 'knowing that' something is the case. Thus a person may build up a considerable bank of facts, theories or ideas about a subject, person or thing, without necessarily having any direct experience of that subject, person or thing. A person, may, for example develop a considerable propositional knowledge about, say, midwifery, without ever necessarily having been anywhere near a woman who is having a baby! Presumably it would be more useful to combine that knowledge with some practical experience, but this does not necessarily have to be the case. This, then, is the domain of propositional knowledge. Obviously it is possible to have propositional knowledge about a great number of subject areas ranging from mathematics to literature or from counselling to social work. Any information contained in books must necessarily be of the propositional sort.

In all traditional 'school' and 'college' type educational enterprises, we rely heavily on propositional knowledge. Propositional knowledge is, after all, the substance of what we find in books and papers and what we are offered in lecturers. It might even be said that much of what we talk about falls into the 'propositional' category although, as we shall see, this is not always the case. When we try to convey rather more personal things, such as how we feel, we find that simply using a string of propositions is not enough. Then, we have to depend to a considerable degree on non-verbal communication and on the other person being able, in some way, to **intuit** what we mean. I suspect that quite a lot of interpersonal communication 'works' at this level.

Practical knowledge

Practical knowledge is knowledge that is developed through the acquisition of skills. Thus driving a car or giving an injection demonstrates practical knowledge, though, equally, so does the use of counselling skills that involve the use of specific verbal and non-verbal behaviours and intentional use of counselling interventions as described above. Practical knowledge is synonymous with Ryle's (1949) concept of 'knowing how'. It is more than mere 'knack': practical knowledge is the substance of a smooth performance of a practical or interpersonal skill. A considerable amount of a health professional's time is taken up with the demonstration of practical knowledge – often, but not always, of the interpersonal sort. Everytime a surgeon performs an operation or a nurse changes a wound dressing, he or she is demonstrating practical knowledge in action.

Practical knowledge is also bound up in work, itself. The process of working allows us not only to learn a set of practical skills but also something more personal – something about ourselves. Joseph Conrad, in *Heart of Darkness*, has his hero, Marlow say this about work:

> I don't like work – no man does – but I like what is in the work, – the chance to find yourself. Your own reality – for yourself, not for others – what no other man can ever know. They can only see the mere show, and never can tell what it really means (Conrad, 1902).

There are hints here, too, of **experiential** knowledge – a concept discussed below.

Traditionally, most educational programmes in schools and colleges have concerned themselves primarily with both propositional and practical knowledge and particularly the former. Thus the 'propositional knowledge' aspect of a person is the aspect that is often held in highest regard. Practical knowledge, although respected, is usually seen as slightly less important than the propositional sort. In this way, the 'self' can become highly developed in one sense – the propositional knowledge aspect – at the expense of being skilled in a practical sense. This division between the relative importance of propositional knowledge and technical skill goes back to Plato's *Republic*. We have, perhaps, always felt 'thinkers' to be somehow more important and, in turn, 'intelligent' than 'doers'. Weill and McGill – in relation to experiential learning – sum up this situation well:

> Although experiential, or experienced-based learning can be regarded as the earliest approach to learning for the human race, the significance and potential of it have not been fully recognized until relatively recently. In the formal education system it has tended to be devalued and regarded as somehow fundamentally inferior to those organized forms of knowledge that have been constructed as subjects or disciplines. The practical and the applied do not tend to have the same status in educational institutions as the academic and the abstract. Academic rigour is a commonplace of classroom discourse, that education should be true to the lived experience of learners is an alien idea. The heritage of Aristotle and Descartes still reigns supreme (Weill and McGill, 1989).

It will be interesting to see, as more and more health care professions move into the higher education and university system, whether or not this accent only on the 'academic' will remain. It seems possible that health care professionals will bring with them a range of practical and interpersonal skills that will become valid parts of the curriculum in the way that 'subjects and disciplines' have in the past.

Experiential knowledge

The domain of experiential knowledge is knowledge gained through direct encounter with a subject, person or thing. It is the subjective and affective nature of that encounter that contributes to this sort of knowledge. Experiential knowledge is knowledge through relationship. Such knowledge is synonymous with Roger's (1983) description of experiential learning and with Polanyi's concept of 'personal' knowledge and 'tacit' knowledge (Polanyi, 1958). If we reflect for a moment we may discover that many of the things that are really important to us belong in this domain. If for example we consider our personal relationships with other people, we discover that what we like or love about them cannot be reduced to a series of propositional statements and the feelings we have for them are vital and part of what is most important in our lives. Most encounters with others contain the seeds of experiential knowledge. It is only when we are so detached from other people that we treat them as objects that no experiential learning can occur.

Not that all experiential knowledge is tied exclusively to relationships with other people. For example, I had considerable propositional knowledge about America before I went there. When I went there, all that propositional knowledge was changed considerably. What I had known was changed by my direct experience of the country. I had developed experiential knowledge of the place. Experiential knowledge is not of the same type or order as propositional or practical knowledge. It is, nevertheless, important knowledge, in that it effects everything else we think about or do.

Experiential knowledge is necessarily personal and idiosyncratic. Indeed, as Rogers (1985) points out, it may be difficult to convey to another person in words. Words tend to be loaded with personal (often experiential) meanings and thus to understand each other we need to understand the nature of the way in which the people with whom we converse use words. It is arguable, however, that such experiential knowledge is sometimes conveyed to others through gesture, eye contact, tone of voice, infection and all the other non-verbal and paralinguistic aspects of communication (Argyle, 1975). Indeed, it may be experiential knowledge that is passed on when two people (for example a health visitor and her client) become very involved with each other in a conversation, a learning encounter or counselling.

As a development of the above discussion of three types of knowledge, it is possible to define experiential learning as **any learning activity that enhances the development of experiential knowledge**. Experiential learning, then, is personal learning: learning that makes a difference to our self concept. As all interpersonal relationships with others, both within and without the health care professions, involve an investment of self, it seems reasonable to argue that any learning methods that involve the self and that involve personal knowledge are likely to enhance personal effectiveness. We cannot, after all, learn interpersonal skills by rote, nor merely by mechanically learning a series of behaviours. We need to spend time reflecting on ourselves and on receiving feedback on our performance from other people.

On the other hand, it should be noted that the concept of 'self' is highly problematic. It is not uncommon for people in the interpersonal skills training field to talk and write about concepts of 'self' and of 'self-awareness'. Given that the 'self' is an abstraction – it is a concept and not a thing – it becomes equally as problematic to talk of 'self-awareness'. While the term 'self' is a useful shorthand for 'person' or for talking about who we are, the danger of reification is always present.

Figure 1.1 illustrates the interplay between the three types of knowledge described in this section. As we have noted, propositional, practical and experiential forms of knowledge do not exist independently of each other. Each needs the other to 'support' it. Also, in relation to the figure, we may note that, at

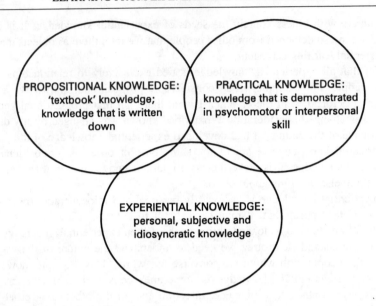

Figure 1.1 Types of knowledge

different times, an individual might use different types of knowledge in different proportions. Thus the person who is undertaking a degree course might find him or herself more caught up in the 'propositional' domain, while the practising clinician may access the 'practical' knowledge domain more frequently. What binds both together, though, is the 'experiential' domain – the domain that 'personalizes' all other types of knowledge.

THE HISTORICAL DEVELOPMENT OF EXPERIENTIAL LEARNING

People have always learned from experience. However, the idea of experiential learning as an educational concept is a relatively recent one. It will be useful to review some of the historical roots of the concept in order to make sense of some of the experiential learning methods that follow in the next chapter.

Drawing on the work of American pragmatic philosopher, John Dewey (1916; 1938), Keeton and Associates (1976) described experiential learning as including learning through the process of living and including work experience, skills developed through hobbies and interests and non-formal educational activities. This approach to definition is reflected in the FEU project report 'Curriculum opportunity' which asserts that, for the purposes of that report, experiential learning referred to the knowledge and skills acquired through life and work experience and study (FEU, 1983).

Pfeiffer and Goodstein (1982) offer a different approach to the concept by describing an 'experiential learning cycle' which spells out the possible process of experiential learning (Figure 1.2) This cycle not only suggests the format for organizing experiential learning but also makes tacit reference to the way in which people learn through experience.

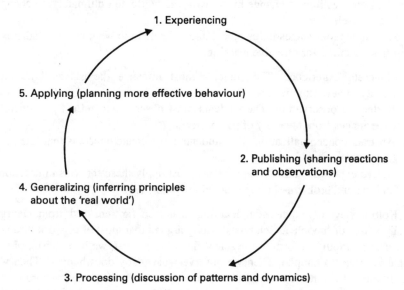

Figure 1.2 Experiential learning cycle (after Pfeiffer and Goodstein, 1982)

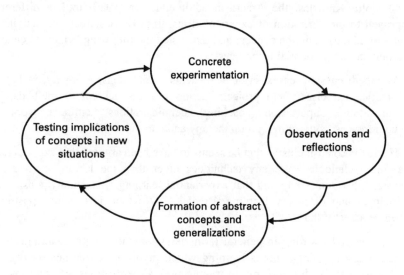

Figure 1.3 Experiential learning cycle (after Kolb, 1994)

Kolb (1984) was more explicit about this learning process in his 'experiential learning model' (Figure 1.3). In this model, concrete experience is the starting point for a reflective process that echoes Paulo Freire's (1972) concept of 'praxis'. Praxis, for Freire is the combination of reflection-and-action-on-the-world: a transforming process that is one of man's distinguishing features and one that enables him to change his view of the world and ultimately, to change the world itself.

Kolb notes four stages in his model and links them to what he calls 'adaptive abilities' required for effective learning:

1. Concrete experience. The students must immerse themselves fully and openly in new experiences.
2. Reflective observation. The students must observe and reflect on concrete experiences from a variety of perspectives.
3. Abstract conceptualization. The students must create concepts that integrate their observations into logical theories.
4. Active experimentation. The students must apply these theories in decision-making and problem-sharing (quoted in Quinn, 1995).

Kolb's view of experiential learning is not so far removed from George Kelly's idea of 'people as scientists'. Kelly argued that most of us work through life using a modified form of the scientific process. First, we hypothesize about what is likely to happen. Then we observe what really does happen. Then we modify our hypothesis in the light of our findings. In this way, according to Kelly, we constantly modify our views and beliefs about the nature of the world (Kelly, 1955).

Malcolm Knowles, the American adult educator (1980) took a different approach to the definition of experiential learning. He described the activities that took place within the concept and thus listed the following, which he called 'participatory experiential techniques':

Group discussion, cases, critical incidents, simulations, role-play, skills practice exercises, field projects, action projects, laboratory methods, consultative supervision (coaching), demonstrations, seminars, work conferences, counselling, group therapy and community development.

His list is so all-inclusive that he seems to have been arguing that experiential learning techniques were any techniques other than the lecture method or private, individual study and that experiential learning was synonymous with participant and discovery learning. Boydel (1976) took just such a position when he asserted that:

Experiential learning in general terms is synonymous with meaningful discovery learning. This is learning which involves the learner sorting things out for himself by restructuring his perceptions of what is happening.

Boydel seems to stress the need for 'discovery' to be 'meaningful' – presumably to the learner in question. It would be possible to argue, for instance, that not all discovery was particularly loaded with meaning. I might discover, for example, that I had weeds growing in part of my lawn but that discovery would not be of great value to me. On the other hand, to discover that when I use a particular tone of voice with patients, they are not particularly encouraged by it, might be of use to me in future encounters with patients. That 'meaning' also helps me to restructure what happens next, i.e. how I talk to patients in the future. On the other hand, the term 'meaningful discovery learning' is a fairly broad one and Boydel qualifies is definition even further when he suggests that experiential learning is 'in general terms' synonymous with it. What, it might be asked, are the terms under which it is not synonymous? Also, the sentence that follows is fairly vague and we might ask whether or not students are ever not 'sorting things out and restructuring their perceptions'.

To summarize the position adopted by those writers who devised their definitions of experiential learning from the work of Dewey would involve noting first the accent on some sort of cycle of events starting with concrete experience. It is worth noting that Kolb's and Pfeiffer and Goodstein's cycles were anticipated by Dewey himself:

> Thinking includes all of these steps, the sense of a problem, the observation of conditions, the formation and rational elaboration of a suggested conclusion and the active experimental testing (Dewey, 1916).

In passing, though, we might note that Dewey is describing, perhaps, a particular type of thinking. Presumably he would not argue that all thinking involves this rather rational series of steps. Daydreaming, for example, might not fulfil Dewey's conditions for thinking.

The notion of learning from experience being a cycle involving action and reflection was a theme frequently echoed among modern writers (see, for example Hampden Turner, 1966; Kelly, 1970). Kolb's notion of transformation of experience and meaning can also be traced back to Dewey. He wrote that:

> In a certain sense every experience should do something to prepare a person for later experiences of a deeper and more expansive quality. That is the very meaning of growth, continuity, reconstruction of experience (Dewey, 1938).

We might, of course, argue that not every experience we have prepares us for later experiences of a 'deeper and more expansive quality'. We might also challenge what is meant by the phrase 'deeper and more expansive' in this connection. It seems likely that a number of our day-to-day experiences are of the 'ordinary' kind that do not, particularly, spur us on to deeper and more expansive experiences. However, if we want to 'grow', in the sense that Dewey seems to be implying, we need to make sure that we notice what happens to us and to notice the experiences that we have. As we have noted, earlier, it is easy simp-ply to allow our lives to 'live us' rather than for us to 'live our lives'. We can, if we are not careful, turn on to 'automatic pilot' rather too easily.

This, then, was the influence on experiential learning from the Dewey perspective. The accent, throughout, was on the primacy of personal experience and on reflection as the tool for changing knowledge and meaning. We have noted, too, that some accounts of experiential learning can involve a rather nebulous use of description and language. This, indeed, may constitute a real difficulty in experiential learning theory: that the language used is imprecise or so **general** as to make identifying a **real theory** from it, impossible. We might note, in passing, that even the word 'experience' is a word that is difficult to pin down with any precision. It is a 'large' word and covers a huge range of possibilities.

The other main influence on the development of experiential learning was the school of psychology known as 'humanistic psychology'. Humanistic psychology developed in the 1940s, '50s and '60s as a reaction to the 'mechanism' of behavioural psychology and the determinism of psychodynamic psychology. It argued that people were free to choose their own lives and thus were 'authors' of their own existence. This philosophical perspective drew heavily on the existentialism of Sartre (1956), Heidegger (1927) and others. Humanistic psychology's main leaders, particularly in the 1960s (which offered exactly the right climate in which humanistic psychology could flourish) were Carl Rogers (1957, 1967, 1975) and Abraham Maslow (1972), who is said to have named humanistic psychology (Grossman, 1985). Rogers is particularly well known for his client-centred counselling and for his student-centred learning methods.

Many of the experiential learning methods described below developed out of the school of humanistic psychology, which, rather like Deweyan educational practices, emphasized the uniqueness of human experience and human interpretation of the world. It should be noted, in passing, that Rogers had been considerably influenced by Dewey as he had been taught at university by a student of Dewey's, William Kilpatrick (Kirschenbaum, 1979). In this way, we begin to develop a sense of experiential learning's heritage: American (although drawing, also, from European philosophical traditions), with a heavy emphasis on personal experience and personal development.

ACQUIRING INTERPERSONAL SKILLS IN THE HEALTH PROFESSIONS: NUMBER 3

Suspending judgment

Notice how an internal censor tends to divide up what other people say into right and wrong. Try suspending judgment on other people until you fully hear what they say. Even then, try to remain non-judgmental! This skill is one of the basic prerequisites of effective counselling.

CHARACTERISTICS OF EXPERIENTIAL LEARNING

Moving on from the above discussion of experiential learning, from the theory of knowledge and from the historical perspective, it is possible to draw out those characteristics that go to make up the approach to learning known as the experiential approach. These characteristics are offered as a further means of clarification and as the beginning of practical guidelines about how to use the approach in practice. In the next chapter, specific experiential learning methods will be described in detail.

In experiential learning there is an accent on action

Both the Dewey and the humanistic approaches to experiential learning involve the learner in action. This is not to say that the learner is 'doing something' in a trivial sense but that she is engaged in an activity that should lead to learning. This is in opposition to traditional teaching/learning strategies that require that the learner remain passive in relation to an active teacher who is the dispenser of knowledge. Freire (1972) has called this traditional approach the 'banking' approach to education: knowledge is delivered to the learner in chunks and the learner later cashes out this information in examinations. The experiential learning approach is closer to Freire's concept of 'problem posing' education. Here, problems are encountered through discussion, argument and action. The learner is no longer passive but in dialogical relationship with an equally active teacher.

There is a second, less important sense, of action too. In experiential learning the learner is often physically moving to take part in structured activities, role play, psychodrama and so on, as opposed to more traditional learning situations in which the learner is sat behind a desk or table. The issue, here, may be one of interest and motivation. It may be the case that when we are involved and active in what we are learning, we find it more interesting and thus learn more readily. After all, in passive lecturing, we are dependent mostly on one stimulus – the voice of the lecturer. When we are active in learning, we experience a multitude of stimuli.

There is also a third sense of action. It may be that we learn best of all when we are actively involved in doing something. We might reflect on the fact that almost all health professionals are involved in actively helping other people. Many students, too, complain of the 'theory/practice' gap – the gap that they perceive to exist between what they are taught in college and what they find when they go into practice. Often, students acknowledge that they 'learn most' from working, directly, in the clinical or practice field (Burnard, 1992). All of this suggests, perhaps, that we learn 'best' when we are not merely passive 'takers in' of knowledge but are working in some way as we learn. This sense of action is, perhaps, illustrated well by the American educator, Lindeman, who wrote:

Learning which is combined with action provides a peculiar and solid enrichment. If, for example, you are interested in art, you will gain much more if you paint as well as look at pictures and read about the history of art. If you happen to be interested in politics, don't be satisfied with being a spectator: participate in political action. If you enjoy nature, refuse to be content with the vicarious experiences of naturalists; become a naturalist yourself. In all these ways, learning becomes an integral part of living until finally the old distinction between life and education disappears. In short, life itself becomes a perpetual experience of learning (Lindeman, 1956).

This sense of the expression is more than simply being interested by being offered a range of stimuli. It is a case of learning though various modes: the muscular and active mode as well as the cognitive mode.

Another commentator highlights, too, the differences between simply taking in knowledge and learning through action:

Much of the learning that takes place in class proceeds through instruction, in which information or knowledge is transmitted from an instructor to the learner, while much of the learning that takes place outside class proceeds through acting (or in some cases, seeing another person act), and then experiencing or observing the consequences of action [emphasis added] (Coleman, 1976).

In a way, this is perhaps the most important sense of action. Throughout our lives, we are compelled to act: as a reaction to the circumstances we find ourselves in, because our jobs and lives dictate it and even as a survival mechanism. If we avoid action, we often find that we suffer anxiety and even depression. It is almost as though action is a major and almost determining mark of being human. Not only that, but it is also a major source of learning. We learn more when we act than when we avoid action: we also get a lot more done!

Learners are encouraged to reflect on their experience

Most writers acknowledge that experience alone is not sufficient to ensure that learning takes place. Importance is placed on the integration of new experience with past experience through the process of reflection (Freire, 1972; Kilty, 1983; Kolb, 1984; Burnard, 1985). Reflection may be an introspective act in which the learner alone integrates new experience with old. It may also be a group process whereby sense is made of an experience through group discussion. If reflection as a group activity is to be successful, the group leader is required to act as a group facilitator and may require special skills and knowledge. These skills and types of knowledge are discussed in later chapters of this book. It is suggested that the skills associated with group facilitation are different to the skills associated with the usual processes of teaching in that the group facilitator takes a non-directive or non-authoritarian stance in relation to the learners. In a reflective group, the leader as facilitator is not ascribing meanings to experience nor offering explanations but allowing learners to do these things for themselves.

In recent years, much has been written about the process of reflection and its value in the training of health care professionals. I feel, though, that a more important issue is that raised by the question: 'can we not reflect?' Just as action seems to be a more or less defining human attribute, so, too, is reflection. It seems rare that we act without any forethought and even rarer that we act without looking back at what we have done – at least to a minimal degree. Perhaps the secret is to increase the amount that we reflect so that conscious reflection becomes second nature. On the other hand, we cannot always afford to reflect, constantly. We have, through pressure of work and life, simply to get on with things. In this case, it may be possible to set aside 'reflective periods' during which we reflect back over what we have done in order to learn. However, I have a suspicion that this is what most of us already do in order to survive.

A phenomenological approach is adopted by the facilitator

Phenomenology may be defined as the description of objects or situations without their being ascribed values, meanings or interpretations. Phenomenology as a philosophy was developed by Husserl (1931) and underpins the philosophical writings of the existentialists (Sartre, 1956; Macquarrie, 1973).

The facilitator who uses a phenomenological approach restricts himself to the use of description as a means of summarizing what a learner has said and enables that learner to invest their own learning with meaning. The 'valuing' process is left to the learner. It is the learner who ascribes meaning to what is going on in the learning environment and the facilitator's meanings are not automatically foisted on the student. Reflecting this phenomenological approach, which eschews interpretation of experience by another person, Carl Rogers (1983) prefers to use the term 'facilitator of learning' rather than the more traditional terms 'teacher' or 'leader'. In using such a descriptor he hoped to remove the connotation of the teacher as expert or authority in the interpretation of experience. In the literature on experiential learning, the term facilitator is often used in preference to the terms teacher, lecturer, tutor or leader.

There is an accent on subjective human experience

Alfred North Whitehead (1933) discussed the problem of 'dead knowledge' and asserted that knowledge kept no better than fish! The experiential approach to learning stresses the evolving, dynamic nature of knowledge. Rather than evoking R. S. Peter's (1972) notion of education as initiation in to particular ways of knowing, it stresses the importance of the learner understanding and creating a view of the world in that learner's own terms. Postman and Weingartner (1969) noted that traditional education assumes a linear model of knowledge in which there is absolute truth and a single fixed reality. Citing anthropological evidence that our language tends to limit our view of reality (Whorf, 1956) and that the means by which subject matter is communicated fundamentally alters the content of that communication, Postman and Weingartner challenge the linear view of education, claiming that learners need to develop the ability to ask critical questions about any so-called 'facts' that are presented to them. They quote Ernest Hemingway in suggesting that all learners should be encouraged to develop 'shockproof crap-detectors'. Arguably, teachers and lecturers have had the 'last word' on knowledge for long enough. If we really aim to educate students, we should be prepared not only for them to challenge us but for our thinking to change in the process too. This may not be easy as students may have been socialized out of the practice of questioning in this way. On this point, Boreham suggests that:

> Educators wishing to promote learning from experience ... have to revive in their students learning styles which may have been discouraged since primary school – learning from experience depends on learning *how to learn* from experience (Boreham, 1987).

One of the facilitators' first tasks, then, may be to show participants in this sort of learning that questioning, criticizing and disagreeing are all acceptable and, indeed, encouraged.

Experiential learning allows for different means of communicating concepts, accounts for 'multiple realities' and invites critical reflection. In this respect, it differs considerably from the traditional model of education and training. The key, it would seem, is communication between 'teacher' and 'student'. And this is appropriate, given that the subject matter of this book is interpersonal skills. If we want to teach interpersonal skills, we must also demonstrate them. This point about communication and about the changing relationship between teachers and students is highlighted by Paulo Freire:

> only through communication can human life hold meaning. The teacher's thinking is authenticated only by the authenticity of the student's thinking. The teacher cannot think for his students, nor can he impose this thoughts on them. Authentic thinking, thinking that is concerned with *reality*, does not take place in ivory-tower isolation, but only in communication (Freire, 1972).

This leads on, precisely, to the next point.

Human experience is valued as a source of learning

The accent in experiential learning, through its variety of learning methods and through its name, is on experience. Learners, as has been noted, are encouraged to reflect on past experiences to plan for future events. In formulating his concept of andragogy (the theory and practice of the education of adults), Malcolm Knowles (1978, 1980) stresses the value of experience in the sphere of adult learning. He maintains that as an individual matures so she accumulates an expanding reservoir of experience that causes her to become a rich resource for learning. Knowles argues that the resource should be tapped in the educational process because, as Knowles puts it: 'To an adult, his experience is who he is' (Knowles, 1978). Thus, for Knowles, there is an important ontological issue: an adult's experience is not something exterior and tacked on but is part of the person's self-concept. Experiential learning then is an attempt to make use of human experience as part of the learning process. It may be noted that the humanistic approach to experiential learning pays particular attention to the emotional aspect of the individual's experience (Heron, 1981).

Only you live your particular life and only you live through the experiences that you have. This leads us to make various assumptions that turn out to be, in varying degrees, the case. First, some of us assume that everyone else around us lives a similar life. This is most noticeable in early childhood. Many people who have had 'odd' childhoods of various sorts will remember believing, in the early days, that 'everyone's life is like this'. It is only as we grow up a little that we begin to appreciate that other children live different sorts of lives. On the other hand, further living may bring us to the conclusion that, looked at broadly, most of us do live similar sorts of lives. We mostly experience love (or lack of it), happiness (and its opposite), enjoyment (and other emotions) and so on. It is, perhaps, only the details that are different. In other words, much of human experience is common to a wide range of people. It is, perhaps, the quality and amount of experiences that differ.

The second assumption that we sometimes make seems to contradict the first. We can find ourselves believing that we are the only ones that have certain experiences. If we have thoughts, feelings and behaviours that do not, at first glance, seem very common, we can quickly assume that we are alone in experiencing them. However, if we look around us and listen to others, we will probably find that most other people do experience the 'odd' thoughts, feelings and behaviours that we have. This idea is put well by Carl Rogers (1967) who suggested that 'what is most personal is most universal'. What I think is uncomfortably unique to me is probably common to you – if only we were both able to openly acknowledge the fact.

Everyone is listened to

Listening, as we shall see in the chapter about counselling in this book, is a vital part of working, interpersonally, with clients and colleagues. In using experiential learning methods, it is vital that the facilitator not only listens to all group members but that he or she also encourages group members to listen to each other. In this respect, too, he or she must act as a role model of excellent listening. People often seem to learn to listen by being listened to. They also learn if they are allowed to explore ideas and voice their opinions – even as those opinions come to them. There is an old saying that 'I don't know what I think until I hear what I say'. If there is any truth in the saying, then we need to be heard in order to sort out what we think. The experiential learning facilitator needs to avoid 'premature closure' in discussions and to make sure everyone gets a chance to 'explore' what they feel about a topic and to verbalize those explorations.

There have been other, useful summaries, of what experiential learning is about. Experiential learning was defined by the Crisis Research and Training Group (Murgatroyd, 1982) as having four main components:

1. the learner is aware of the processes which are taking place, and which are enabling learning to occur;
2. the learner is involved in a reflective experience which enables the person to relate current learning to past, present and future, even if these time relationships are felt rather than thought;
3. personally significant experience and content: what is being learned and how it is being learned hold a special importance for that person;
4. there is an involvement of the whole self – body, thoughts, feelings and actions, not just of the mind; in other words, the learner is engaged as a whole person (Murgatroyd, 1982).

Meanwhile, Woolfe has summarized what he considers to be 'concrete propositions' about the nature and application of experiential learning and these serve as a useful summary of many of the points raised in this chapter:

- Experiential learning is concerned with the experience of individuals, not just with their participation. Participants are asked to consider and utilize their own experience as a basis for self-understanding and assessment of their own needs, resources and objectives.
- The individual participant is regarded as an active rather than a passive participant in the process of defining and putting into practice rather than a passive participant in the process of defining and putting into practice educational agendas and methodologies.
- Through this process, power (locus of control) is shifted away from the teaching in the direction of the learner. Another way to put this would be to say that the nature of the teacher-student relationship is usually asymmetrical; the former has more power than the latter ... [in the experiential learning approach] this asymmetry is reduced. Learners are planning, carrying out and evaluating their own learning. The 'expert' and the learner engage in a process that is concerned not with the former transferring facts into the latter but rather with facilitating an active process of learning in the student. It could be described as a move away from the model for education in which the learner is seen as an empty vessel to be filled full of facts towards one in which the latter is seen as a candle to be lit; a potential to be developed.

- The participant becomes responsible for his or her own learning. The expert is a resource and a provider of structure, but learning is seen as taking place when the learner is trying actively to assimilate external knowledge into his or her own internal frame reference (Woolfe, 1992).

Finally, while discussing the characteristics of experiential learning it may be noted that what is under consideration is:

1. a set of teaching/learning methods and
2. an attitude towards learning.

What is **not** under discussion, however, is the idea of experiential learning as a **formal learning theory**. As far as the author has been able to ascertain, experiential learning has never been offered as a learning theory in the way, for instance, that **social learning theory** has. Rather, it is a way of thinking about teacher and facilitator attitudes, programme planing and about a general orientation towards teaching and learning.

The limits of personal experience and of experiential learning

As with any approach to learning, there are limitations to experiential learning. First, though, the question of the limits of personal experience. First, we cannot experience everything. It is self-evident that no one has enough time, the physical and psychological attributes or the desire to experience everthing that it is possible to experience. To that extent, then, we must rely on the evidence from others. Second, simply to experience a situation for the sake of it may be another form of time wasting. We can also learn vicariously – by observing others and by listening to the experience of others. Most traditional education is based, in some ways, on this approach. After all, the contents of books and lecturers are, by necessity, made of other people's experiences. It would be odd, indeed, to reject all of these, 'other people's' experiences. This is particularly true, of course, of research-based experience. It seems reasonable to assume that to gather evidence from a wide range of people is in some ways more useful that simply relying on our own experience. The point of the discussion of experiential learning, in this chapter, is not in any way to deny the validity of other people's experiences but simply to offer an alternative approach. There is no reason at all why experiential learning activities should not sit alongside more formal, lecture-based approaches in health care curricula. Indeed, this mix is likely to be an appropriate one for, in the end, we do not all learn in the same sorts of ways. Some people, perhaps, learn more from a series of lectures, followed by reflection on their own experience, than they do from a series of role plays. As in most things, a sense of balance is called for.

Second, not everyone likes experiential learning activities. This is a slightly complicated issue. It would be difficult to claim that all educational activities must be ones that are popular with students. It seems likely that most people will have a favourite or preferred way of learning and be less motivated by other ways. The point about experiential learning methods, however, is their personal nature. By definition, they involve students in sharing their ideas, reflections and even their emotions with each other. Just as not everyone likes to get angry or to cry in public, not everyone likes to express themselves 'publicly' in a classroom or lecture theatre. As Sidney Jourard's (1964) research has indicated, people vary in their ability and desire to self-disclose. It would seem difficult to put up an educational argument for forcing self-disclosure and, in practice, the enterprise would presumably be a failure. For no one, in the end, is going to disclose that which they do not choose to.

There is, however, a dilemma. If we considered a 'worst possible' case, in which all students in a group chose not to take part in experiential learning activities, we would be faced with the issue of how best to teach interpersonal skills at all. In practice, this sort of situation is unlikely to arise and is certainly unknown to the author. In my experience, if students are introduced to experiential learning activities slowly and not asked to reveal things about themselves or to self-disclose too quickly, then they are usually happy to take part. As we have seen, part of the issue is the modelling of certain attitudes and values by the facilitator. If the facilitator can be encouraging and accepting to his or her students, then it seems likely that those students are likely to be happier in taking part in experiential learning activities. There will, however, always be the exception. And in my view, no one should be forced to take part in any educational activity. This means that, very occasionally, other sorts of educational experiences will have to be arranged for single or small groups of students.

In the next chapter we will consider the range of experiential learning methods. The experiential learning approach as an attitude commends a model of education that stresses autonomous judgement, freedom of thought and the value of subjective human experience – values that may be supported by anyone working in the health professions.

Experiential learning methods for acquiring interpersonal skills | 2

EXPERIENTIAL LEARNING METHODS

A wide variety of learning methods have evolved, often out of the humanistic approach to the field, that have come to be known as 'experiential learning methods'. All of those methods focus on the student or learner being offered an experience, followed by the reflection and making sense of that experience that was described in Chapter 1. In this chapter, some of those methods are examined critically and practical suggestions are offered for their use in interpersonal skills training. The methods differ from more traditional teaching methods (which usually involve some sort of 'telling' on the part of the teacher). Experiential learning methods all honour the principles of experiential learning discussed in the previous chapter.

PAIRS EXERCISES

Pairs exercises, such as the ones described in the last chapter of this book are particularly useful for learning and practising interpersonal skills such as counselling skills. The usual format for the pairs exercise is that each person nominates themselves A or B. Then A practises the particular skill (for example, using open-ended questions) in the supportive presence of B. After a period in these roles, the two people swap round and B practises the skill in the supportive presence of A. It is important that the exercise is not seen as a form of conversation but as a highly structured learning exercise. After each of the individuals has had a turn in the driving seat, the pair may spend time freely evaluating and appraising the exercise. Alternatively, the pair may rejoin a larger group to discuss the exercise with other people. The format is illustrated in Figure 2.1.

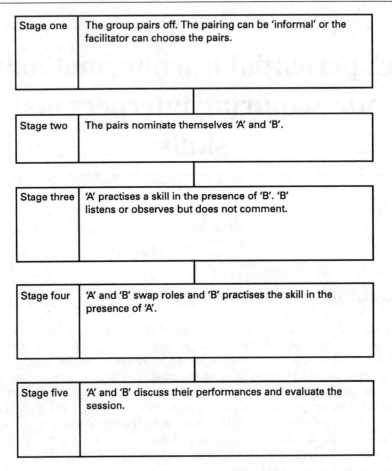

Stage one	The group pairs off. The pairing can be 'informal' or the facilitator can choose the pairs.
Stage two	The pairs nominate themselves 'A' and 'B'.
Stage three	'A' practises a skill in the presence of 'B'. 'B' listens or observes but does not comment.
Stage four	'A' and 'B' swap roles and 'B' practises the skill in the presence of 'A'.
Stage five	'A' and 'B' discuss their performances and evaluate the session.

Figure 2.1 Format for pairs exercises

An alternative use of the pairs format is for the pair in question to take a theme and for one person to discuss that theme while the other person listens. After a prescribed time, the pair switch roles and the listener becomes the talker and vice versa. After an equal amount of time in this second phase of the activity, the pair may link up with another pair and discuss the issue in a foursome. Alternatively, they may be invited back into a larger group to discuss the issues in among all of their colleagues. Suitable themes and questions, related to health care and interpersonal skills development, include the following:

- What do I need to do to enhance my interpersonal skills?
- In what respects am I interpersonally skilled?
- What do I need to do to improve my counselling skills?
- What am I like as a teacher?

- What are my personal strengths/weaknesses?
- How well do I conduct interviews?
- How do my colleagues see me?
- How do my family see me?
- What are the best and worst things about my relationships with my clients?
- What are my strengths and weaknesses as a social worker/nurse/doctor etc.

Examples of the use of the pairs method in health care training:

- physiotherapy: practising introducing self to new patients;
- GPs: rehearsing terminating a consultation;
- speech therapy: practising offering and explaining new information to children.

STRUCTURED GROUP ACTIVITIES

Structured group exercises allow for the experiential learning cycle to be worked through by a learning group. There are a number of publications (including this one) which describe a variety of group activities for enhancing interpersonal, social and counselling skills (Burnard, 1985; Murgatroyd, 1986). The idea of these activities is that the group undertakes an experience after which they discuss their thoughts and feelings about the experience and apply the new learning to the real or clinical situation. The adventures of this approach include the sharing of a common experience, the generation of a wide range of possible solutions to practical problems and the realization of both the personal and the common nature of group experience. Much can be learnt, experientially, about how to run and be members of groups by taking part in structured group activities. Many of the best structured group activities are those that the facilitator or the group devise themselves.

There are some important guidelines that may help in the smooth running of structured group activities that may be identified as follows:

- full and clear instructions must be given to the group and questions asked by the facilitator to establish that everyone in the group is clear about what to do;
- participation should always be voluntary and participants given the chance to sit out as observers;
- plenty of time must be set aside after the exercise in order to 'process' or discuss the activity; rushed processing of activities is a sure sign of an inexperienced facilitator;
- the facilitator should be just that and not rush to offer his or her own explanations or interpretations of what has just happened in the group;
- a debriefing period should follow the exercise to allow time for the participants to re-enter their normal, everyday roles;
- the facilitator should encourage the group members to link any new learning with 'real life' and with their jobs away from the group. Group members should also be encouraged to practice any new skills learned, as soon as possible.

Examples of the use of structured group exercises in health care training

- nursing: developing self-awareness in mental health nursing;
- social work: learning counselling skills;
- probation officers: learning appropriate assertiveness.

ACQUIRING INTERPERSONAL SKILLS IN THE HEALTH PROFESSIONS: NUMBER 4

Naive phenomenology

This refers to the notion of suspending the development of theories. As we go through life, especially if we have had a psychological, sociological or political training, we tend to theorize about what we or other people are doing. Try, for a period, merely to observe other people and resist the temptation to slot what they do into a particular theory. This activity can help to sharpen up observational skills and help to improve descriptive ability. It does not, of course, have any predictive power!

ROLE-PLAY

Role-play involves the setting up of an imagined and possible situation, acting out that situation and learning from the drama (Figure 2.2). More specifically, the cycle indicates that after a role-play, a period of reflection is necessary, followed by feedback from other participants in order that new learning can be absorbed from the drama.

The first stage of a successful role-play, 'setting the scene', consists of inviting a number of participants to play out a scene, either from their own past or one they are likely to encounter in the future. Scenes replayed from the past are useful in that the role-play allows further reflection on those past situations. Anticipated scenes, on the other hand, allow for the rehearsal of new behaviour.

Once the 'players' have been selected, scenery and props of a simple sort should be used to create the invoked scene, for example, tables and chairs, suitably arranged.

Once scenery has been set and roles cast, the role-play can begin. The facilitator acts as 'director' and helps the actors to fully exploit their roles. Occasionally the facilitator may stop the role-play and allow a character to slow down her acting or take time out to consider how best to play the next part of the scene.

When the scene has been played out to the satisfaction of the players, the facilitator asks the players to reflect on their performances and those of their colleagues. An appropriate feedback order is as follows:

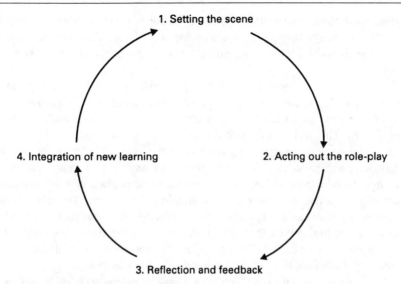

Figure 2.2 The stages involved in role-play

1. The principle actor self-reports on her performance.
2. The supporting actors offer the principle actor feedback on her performance.
3. The audience offers the principal actor feedback on her performance.
4. Those three stages are repeated for all the other actors.

Following such feedback (which takes considerable time and should not be hurried), the role-play can be re-run and new learning, gained from the feedback, can be incorporated into the new performance.

Role-play is particularly useful for teaching and learning in the following domains of interpersonal skills training:

- counselling skills training (Nelson-Jones, 1981);
- group facilitation training (Heron, 1973);
- assertiveness training (Alberti and Emmons, 1982);
- social skills rehearsal (Ellis and Whittington, 1981).

Apart from the use of role-play in the development of interpersonal skills, it may also be used as an aid to developing empathy; to rehearse initial practitioner/client meetings; to develop interview skills; to practise public speaking or the delivery of seminar papers and as a problem-solving activity. In this later context, a problem situation is acted out with a variety of possible 'solutions'. The actors and the audience decide which solution feels best after they have completed the various role-plays.

What, then, are the limitations of role-play? The first limitation is that, by definition, role-play is never real, it is always a simulation of a real situation.

Unlike most other experiential activities, the participants are always asked to act either as though they were someone else or as though they were in a situation other than the present one. Some sense of the artificial will always be present.

Indeed, it can be argued that if this slight sense of unreality is not present, then the role-play is not working. If the situation cannot be distinguished from real life then the actors are no longer acting; they are reacting realistically in present time. This is fine as far as it goes, but it is not role-play.

A question mark must always hang over the issue of whether or not the behaviour participants exhibit in role-play bears any relation to the behaviour that they would exhibit in 'real life'. A role-play takes place in a safe environment – very often in a college or a training department. The players are supported by their colleagues who watch knowing that what they see is play acting. In real life, neither the safe environment nor the supportive colleagues would necessarily be there. Who is to say if what someone does in a role-play is in any way equivalent to what that person would do away from it?

Just as we would not expect actors in a play to extend their roles into their lives away from the theatre, so we cannot guarantee any necessary continuity between performances in a role-play and performance in the real health care setting. Acting is, after all, acting.

The second limitation is that role-play may appeal only to those who are extrovert enough to take part in it. It seems likely that those who observe the role-play gain considerably from looking on, through vicarious learning, but there is no substitute for taking part. Acting, however, does not appeal to everyone. Some participants may be unable to enter into a role or have no particular wish to do so. While such reservations must be honoured by the facilitator, they must call into question the validity of the method.

Another more complicated limitation may also arise here. The anxious-to-please participant or unassertive participant may agree to take part in order to please the facilitator. Alternatively, such a participant may feel compelled to take part because of group pressure. It is naive to think that all the facilitator has to do is tell the group that no one has to take part and that the decision by a participant not to take part will be fully honoured. Group dynamics and individual psychologies are more complex than that. The need to please the facilitator or other group members may override individual needs and wants.

Finally, comes the question of transfer of learning. It has been acknowledged that role-play can never be real life. It is always an approximation, a symbolic representation. Can we assume, therefore, that the skills developed through role-play necessarily transfer over into the real health care setting? One may hope that they do but such hope can never amount to a guarantee. What we are asking is that skills learned in an artificial setting be used in a real setting. It may just be that the disjunction between the artificial and the real is too great.

It is important to differentiate between role-play and skills rehearsal. Role-play, as we have seen, involves inviting people to play out roles other than their own. Skills rehearsal, on the other hand, is where skills such as counselling and group facilitation are practised but with the person remaining who she is in present time. A typical example of skills rehearsal is the pairs exercise format, described above. Thus a pairs exercise which develops listening skills through one person consciously giving her attention to another while the other talks is skills rehearsal. It is not role-play. This important difference is sometimes blurred. The criticisms that may be levelled at role-play are not necessarily true of skills rehearsal.

These then are some of the limitations of role-play. Having stated them it is important to acknowledge, also, that used wisely, role-play remains a useful method of activity involving participants in their own learning. If it is necessary to 'try out' new behaviours and new skills before working in the field (and it seems difficult to argue otherwise), role-play offers a valuable vehicle for such practice. What are offered now are some practical guidelines for running role-plays.

Role-play is rather different to structured group exercises, in that in a role-play, the participants are invited to enter different roles to their normal ones and to try out new behaviour. It is helpful if participants volunteer for particular roles. Definite stages in the role-play process may be identified as follows:

1. Explanation, by the facilitator of the aims of the role-play. Sometimes this aim is negotiated within the group or identified as likely to be useful, by a small number of group members.
2. Agreement about roles to be played out.
3. Outlining of possible scripts. This stage is optional: some groups prefer to 'ad lib' the role-play.
4. The acting out of the role-play.
5. Evaluation of their performances by the main characters in the role-play.
6. Evaluation of the performances by any 'observers' in the group (those members not directly taking part in the role-play).
7. Discussion and processing of the role-play with a full discussion of how everyone felt.
8. If required, a re-enactment of the role-play to allow for changes in performance. This is particularly useful in assertiveness groups and counselling skills groups, where brand new skills are being rehearsed. The second performance can often allow performers to add to their skills by taking account of the discussion generated by the first role-play.

Examples of the use of role-play in health care training

- social work: preparing to work with abused children;
- GPs: anticipating counselling depressed patients;
- occupational therapy: practising planning rehabilitation with patients.

ACQUIRING INTERPERSONAL SKILLS IN THE HEALTH PROFESSIONS: NUMBER 5

Practising new behaviour

Try something new! Mostly we think of ourselves as only having a limited repertoire of behaviours because we have a certain, rather fixed, view of ourselves. In trying out a new way of acting and even trying out exaggerated behaviour, we may learn something about our self-imposed limitations. The novelist, Kurt Vonnegut, once wrote: 'We are what we pretend to be ...' (Vonnegut, 1969). Try pretending to be something different! This activity may be used in a group context and group participants may be encouraged to try out new behaviours for the duration of the workshop. Some people are suprised how easy it is to be different!

PSYCHODRAMA

A variant of role-play is psychodrama (Moreno, 1959; 1969; 1977). In psychodrama, a 'real life' situation that has been lived by one or more of the group members is re-enacted and then discussed by those actors and by the group. The above stages are worked through in psychodrama in much the same ways as they are in standard role-play. Slight variations in approach may be noted, however, and the following stages offer a more complete guide to the process of psychodrama:

1. the scene to be replayed is selected;
2. the main 'actor', who has described the scene to be re-enacted, chooses fellow actors, from the group, to play other parts;
3. the main actor briefs those actors about their roles and gives them a clear outline of what happened in the real situation;
4. the psychodrama scene is played out; as it is, the main actor may stop the action to suggest small changes in performance; the aim is to recreate the past scene as completely as possible;
5. the performance is then processed by the group of actors and ideas are offered by any 'onlookers'.
6. after the discussion, the situation is replayed **as the main actor would have liked it to have occurred**. This is a vital part of psychodrama, that it allows a second chance at playing out a situation and an opportunity for trying out new skills in a 'real' situation. Again, psychodrama is particularly useful for encouraging the development of assertiveness and counselling skills. It may also be used for exploring group members' personal life problems. In this context, however, it should be used with caution and preferably only by

someone experienced in the medium. Both psychodrama and role-play can invoke considerable emotion in both players and observers.

Examples of the use of the psychodrama in health care training

- voluntary workers: helping in deciding when to 'refer on' to other health professionals;
- nursing: reflecting on working with dying patients and bereaved relatives;
- physiotherapy: enhancing performance when working with severely injured young people.

BRAINSTORMING

The process known as 'brainstorming' has frequently been cited as an example of a student-centred or experiential learning method (Heron, 1973; Pfeiffer and Jones, 1974; Kilty, 1983; Brandes and Phillips, 1984).

The basic method of brainstorming may be described as follows. The learning group is encouraged to consider a particular topic and to call out words that they associate with it. These words are then collated on to either a black or white board or onto a series of flip-chart sheets. If the sheets are used they can be hung around the room to form a series of posters that serve as memory aids. During this initial process of calling out of associations, the group is encouraged not to discount any association – often the more bizarre ones can lead to creative thinking (Koberg and Bagnall, 1981).

This process of encouraging associations can be a short one, taking, perhaps, up to five or ten minutes, or it can evolve into a lengthy session of up to forty minutes, as a means of investigating a topic in depth. The noting down of associations in this way can be an end in itself. The activity can lead into a discussion or a more formal lesson. In this sense, brainstorming is used as a warm-up activity to encourage initial thought about a topic.

A further elaboration of the process so far described is for the facilitator or tutor to work through the lists of words, with the group, crossing out obviously inappropriate words. This is more difficult than it sounds! Often what seems inappropriate to one person is important to another!

Following this second process, the facilitator can then work through the lists again, with the group, in order to 'prioritize' items. Prioritizing is the process of putting the items into some sort of rank order. This may mean that the items are sorted along a dimension of 'most appropriate' words to 'least appropriate' words. Out of this activity can arise the subject matter for a discussion or a more formal session. The prioritized list that emerges from this activity can serve as a programme for the next session.

Another method of prioritizing is to invite group members to examine the lists and to place a pre-determined number of ticks against items that interest them most. Again, this method can be used to organize the next part of the programme or to determine the subject matter for the rest of the day, week, or workshop.

This, then, is the basic method of brainstorming with various slight additions to make its use more extensive. The approach described above may be used in various ways. First, as we have seen, it can be used as a method of determining the content of a course. It can be used at the beginning of a workshop or on the first day of a block of training. Used this way it ensures that the course is truly grounded in the needs and wants of the students. In this way, too, it draws upon students' prior knowledge and experience and may therefore be described as an experiential learning method (Hanks *et al.*, 1977).

Second, the basic method may be used as a problem-solving device (Koberg and Bagnall, 1981; OUCWCG, 1987). Faced with a particular clinical or practical problem in a group discussion, the facilitator may use the brainstorming approach to identify a wide range of ways of solving the problem. Again, this method calls upon the learner's prior experience and it can encourage the reinforcement of learning through practical application. It can also encourage assertive behaviour in that learners see their solutions written up in front of them as viable propositions.

Third, the basic method can be used as an evaluation device. At the end of a workshop or block the group is encouraged to identify their associations regarding what they have learned. These can be identified under headings such as 'knowledge' and 'skills'. Again, the process of prioritizing through the use of participants' ticks can be used to identify the degree of agreement on areas of learning. The outcome of this use of brainstorming can be that new material is identified for the next learning session.

If the method is used as an evaluative process, it is important that plenty of time is set aside for the activity. In this way all aspects of learning can be identified. If the process is rushed, only the very obvious and superficial aspects of learning will surface.

Used in this way, brainstorming becomes a joint evaluation/assessment process: evaluation, in that it encourages a value to be placed on what has been learned so far; assessment, in that it identifies new areas for programme planning. The process is also clearly student-centred. It encourages the learners to identify what they have learned without the tutor's anticipating particular areas of learning. It is worth noting, however, Patton's (1982) point that evaluation and assessment carried out in this way needs to be a very structured activity if it is not to degenerate into a 'free for all'. The tutor using this approach to evaluation needs to consider their level of skills in group facilitation in order to ensure that the evaluation is both systematic and effective.

Another way of using brainstorming is to consider it a method of exploring feelings – the affective domain. Much has been written recently about the need for health professionals to develop self-awareness (Burnard, 1985; Bond, 1986; Jenkins, 1987). Part of this self-awareness development comes through identifying how we feel about something. Thus, brainstorming can become a self-awareness instrument. Two examples of its use in this way can be described.

First, it can be used as a spontaneous activity during a more formal learning session. Thus, during a session on caring for the dying person, the tutor can gently encourage the group to brainstorm their feelings about the topic. Out of such a session can arise areas of personal difficulty or interest and these issues can be used as topics for further discussion. Disclosure of feeling states can also enhance self-awareness (Jourard, 1964; 1971).

Second, it can be used more directly as an 'affective activity' in its own right. Thus, the tutor sets out to explore with the group their feelings about a particular topic. For example, a group of psychiatric nursing students considering the topic of depression may be asked to identify their own feelings from when they have felt depressed. Again, by drawing upon the student's own past experience, used this way, brainstorming is an excellent example of an experiential learning method. This particular format is useful for exploring more 'personal' aspects of the curriculum: spirituality, sexuality, interpersonal relationships, value and belief systems and so forth.

Finally, two variants of the basic method of brainstorming may be considered. One, is the use of brainstorming as a small group activity (Newble and Cannon, 1987). Students are invited to form into small groups of three to five members. In each group, a facilitator or chairperson is elected and that person serves as the one who writes down the associations on flip-chart sheets. After a period of about 15 minutes, the small groups re-form and a plenary session is held. In this session, each group pins up their sheets and all other participants are invited to view the displayed sheets. Out of this viewing period evolves a discussion of a more general sort. The advantage of this approach to brainstorming is that it allows almost everyone to take part. Students who are more reticent in a large group may feel more comfortable working in the small.

The second variant on the basic approach is that of 'individual' brainstorming. Here, students are encouraged to sit quietly on their own and to write down all the associations that they make on a particular topic. When a given period of time has passed (usually between five and ten minutes), those students may be invited to form a plenary session. In this session, two things may be done. One, is to discuss the process of the activity, i.e. what it felt like to carry out the activity. Second, is to invite students to share what they have written down. This, again, must be a voluntary activity. Some of the jottings may be of a personal nature and group members may or may not wish to share them with the whole group.

Used in this way, the process of brainstorming becomes akin to the process of free-association – the basic activity of psychoanalysis (Hall, 1954; Bullock and Stallybrass, 1977). Perhaps because of this, strong feelings may, again, be identified. Again, it is recommended that tutors using this method develop skills in handling emotions. It should, of course, be emphasized that this form of brainstorming is only similar to one aspect of psychoanalysis. Clearly it is nothing to do with psychoanalysis itself in that psychoanalysis is a structured and lengthy therapeutic process that involves interpretation, by a trained analyst, of the associations made by the client. It is not suggested that brainstorming should evolve into a form of do-it-yourself psychoanalysis!

Certain principles emerge out of all the different sorts of brainstorming activities described here and out of the literature cited above. They may be enumerated as follows:

1. Keep it simple but keep it structured. Instructions need to be given clearly and be easily understood. The structure of the activity serves to keep that activity focused.
2. Keep to time. If the activity overruns it may appear loose and unstructured. If it underruns, it may appear rushed.
3. Ensure that all associations are written down exactly as they are offered by the students. It is important that the tutor does not offer an 'interpretation' of students' offerings.
4. Allow everyone to have their say. It is important that domination by one student is kept to a minimum and that all feel free to talk.

Examples of the use of brainstorming in health care training

Brainstorming has wide application in almost all teaching and learning situations. It is particularly useful in identifying individual student groups' reactions to various situations, such as:

- working with people with learning difficulties;
- coping with bereavement;
- feelings about patients or clients' sexuality;
- identifying career moves or prospects.

ACQUIRING INTERPERSONAL SKILLS IN THE HEALTH PROFESSIONS: NUMBER 6

Noticing non-verbal behaviour

Simply, notice the link, or sometimes the lack of it, between what people say and their non-verbal behaviour. Which is 'correct' – the verbal or the non-verbal? Probably the only way to find out is to ask them. Notice whether or not you are consistent in your use of non-verbal behaviour.

THE EXPERIENTIAL LECTURE

Quinn (1995) describes the experiential lecture as a short lecture that precedes an experiential learning session:

This form of lecture is used prior to experiential learning activities and is intended to give participants basic concepts and explanations about the issues in question. For example, a nurse teacher may plan to teach students about self-awareness and may begin with an experiential lecture that provides a theoretical framework for the various activities that follow. Such a framework could consist of the various components of the 'self', the formation of the self-picture, and a review of the methods of gaining greater self-awareness (Quinn, 1995).

It is useful to consider the **format** of an experiential learning session and Figure 2.3 illustrates one approach to organization.

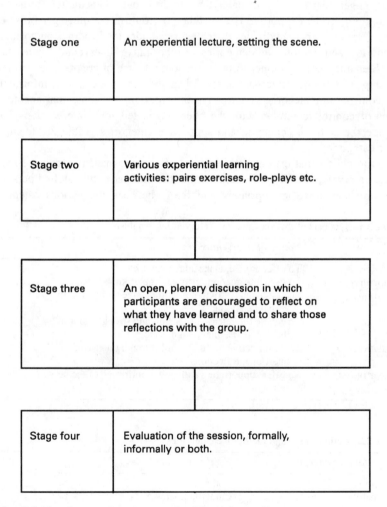

Stage one	An experiential lecture, setting the scene.
Stage two	Various experiential learning activities: pairs exercises, role-plays etc.
Stage three	An open, plenary discussion in which participants are encouraged to reflect on what they have learned and to share those reflections with the group.
Stage four	Evaluation of the session, formally, informally or both.

Figure 2.3 Plan for organizing an experiential training session

SIX CATEGORY INTERVENTION ANALYSIS

Six Category Intervention Analysis (Heron, 1986) developed out of previous work by Blake and Mouton (1972). It is a device for identifying possible types of effective interpersonal interventions between practitioners and clients of various sorts. It is also particularly useful as an interpersonal training tool.

The categories identified in Heron's category analysis are: prescriptive, informative, confronting, cathartic, catalytic and supportive. To be prescriptive is to offer advice or make suggestions. To be informative is to offer information or instruction. To be confronting is to challenge the person's behaviour, attitudes or beliefs. To be cathartic is to enable the release of tension and strong emotion (tears, anger, fear etc.). To be catalytic is to draw out, to encourage further self exploration. To be supportive is to validate or confirm the other person's self-worth. Heron further subdivides the categories under the headings authoritative categories and facilitative categories. Authoritative interventions are those which enable the practitioner to maintain some degree of control over the relationship ('I tell you', interventions), and include the prescriptive, informative and confronting categories. Facilitative interventions are those that enable the locus of control to remain with the client ('you tell me', interventions), and include the cathartic, catalytic and supportive categories. Table 2.1 identifies these categories.

Heron claims that the category analysis offers an exhaustive range of therapeutic interventions. He further claims that the interpersonally skilled person is one who can move appropriately and freely between the various categories

Table 2.1 Synopsis of the Six Category Intervention Analysis

Category	Nature of intervention
Prescriptive	To offer advice, make suggestions etc.
Informative	To give information, instruct, impart knowledge etc.
Confronting	To challenge restrictive or compulsive verbal or non-verbal behaviour.
Cathartic	To enable the release of tension and strong emotion through tears, angry sounds etc.
Catalytic	To be reflective, to 'draw out' through the use of questions, reflections etc.
Supportive	To offer support, be validating, confirming of the person's self-worth.

Table 2.2 Authoritative and facilitative categories

Authoritative categories	Facilitative categories
Prescriptive	Cathartic
Informative	Catalytic
Confronting	Supportive

when using the category analysis as a means of guiding therapeutic action. Heron suggests that no category is more or less important than any other category. Paradoxically, however, he argues that catalytic interventions form a 'bedrock' type of intervention that may serve as the basis for effective communication and counselling. He also offers the view that because we live in a 'non-cathartic society' (Heron, 1977a), where the overt expression of strong emotion is not highly valued, the cathartic category will tend to be less frequently and less skilfully used by many practitioners. Fielding and Llewelyn (1987) also note that there are different degrees of resistance to the overt expression of emotion within the U.K., influenced by culture. Heron goes on to make a case for the therapeutic value of cathartic release – a highly pertinent and contentious argument but one that is beyond the remit of this book. Suffice to say that other commentators may not view cathartic release as being of such importance. George Kelly, for example, in acknowledging the need to 'look forward' in life, rather than to look back at past traumas, says 'the only valid way to live one's life is to get on with it' (Kelly, 1969).

The category analysis is pitched at the level of intention. That is to say that it does not pick out a range of specific verbal behaviours but attempts to guide the user's intentions in making therapeutic interventions. Thus it is in no sense a mechanical, behavioural training device but a means of enabling the user to discriminate between a range of varied therapeutic (and, by implication, non-therapeutic) interventions. The question remains, however, as to the degree to which trainers can have access to people's intentions and whether or not people can remember their intentions, after the event! The word 'intervention' is used, here, to describe any verbal or non-verbal statement or behaviour that the practitioner may use in the therapeutic relationship. The word 'category' is used, here, to denote a range of related interventions.

Heron's analysis offers a starting point for training and research into interpersonal skills. Like all theoretical frameworks, it remains open to revision in the light of experience and research. It is also important to note that Heron's category analysis is not a behavioural analysis in the sense that it breaks down interpersonal skills into microskills. Instead, it aims at identifying people's intentions when engaging in interaction. This analysis of intentions must pose difficulties when attempting to quantify people's views of what they are doing when they engage in human interaction. The whole issue of intentionality is a difficult one and some of the problems in this field are discussed elsewhere (Searle, 1983).

The category analysis can be used in the following ways:

• as a means of identifying therapeutic interventions in counselling, teaching, group work and management;
• as a method of appreciating the range of therapeutic intervention;
• as a training tool: interventions in each of the six categories can be rehearsed in interpersonal skills training as a means of developing competence;

- as a research tool: the author has used the category analysis as a means of helping nurses to identify their strengths and weaknesses throughout the range of categories.

In a recent piece of research which used the analysis as a self-rating scale (Burnard and Morrison, 1988), in a study of more than 80 trained nurses, it was found that most of those nurses perceived themselves as being more skilled in being prescriptive, informative and supportive and least skilled in being catalytic, cathartic and confronting. The study was repeated with a larger group of student nurses and the same profile emerged (Morrison and Burnard, 1988). Heron (1977b) anticipated that health care professionals would be more skilled in the prescriptive, informative and supportive categories and less skilled in being catalytic, cathartic or confronting.

- As an evaluative tool for determining effectiveness across a wide range of therapeutic interventions.

Examples of Six Category Intervention Analysis in health care training

- social work and nursing: Learning counselling skills;
- voluntary workers: Learning telephone counselling skills;
- physiotherapy: Working with patients' emotion release.

These are a range of experiential learning methods that have wide application in the field of interpersonal skills training in the health professions. In later chapters we will consider how best such methods may be used, how to set them up, how to plan their use in a curriculum and how to evaluate their effectiveness as instruments of learning. Before that, it will be helpful to consider the range of interpersonal skills that may be useful to all health professionals.

Interpersonal skills described | 3

The idea of 'interpersonal skills' arises as an answer to the human question: 'here is another person ... what do I do?' The need for interpersonal skills in health professionals is clear and easily articulated: we need them in order to get on with others and to help them. As Martin Buber (1958) is at length to point out: we exist as selves-in-relation: we need other people as much as they need us. Not to be interpersonally skilled as a health care professional is to be ineffective as a health care professional. If you did not believe that interpersonal skills are important, it is doubtful that you would be reading this book.

The range of what constitutes interpersonal skills is vast. A short list of such skills would include at least the following: counselling, group membership skills, assertiveness, social skills, interviewing skills of various sorts, writing skills, using the telephone and group facilitation skills. Examples of how such skills are used in the health care setting are also numerous and a few would include the following:

- counselling skills: talking to the distressed or depressed client, discussing work issues with a colleague;
- assertiveness skills: coping with the 'difficult' client, working within a bureaucracy.

While these are the ones that are described in more detail in this chapter, other, even more 'commonplace' ones should be noted. These might include, at least, the following:

- introductions: the process of identifying ourselves to clients, patients and colleagues is an important skill;
- seeking information: all health professionals have to collect and collate information from patients and clients – both as part of an initial, assessment process and as part of on-going care;
- giving information: being able to help patients, clients and colleagues to appreciate what is wrong with them, what they need to do and how they need to act in the future, is all part of delivering high-quality care;

- listening to patients/clients/colleagues/others: this is probably the most important interpersonal skills of all and one that is returned to frequently in this and other books;
- holding conversations with clients/colleagues/others: easy to overlook, the fact that we need to be able to be 'natural' and to talk to clients and colleagues in an 'everyday' sense is also a skill; most of us learn it but many of us, perhaps, could be better at it;
- enjoying the company of others: rather like holding conversations, the business of simply being with others is an important act;
- breaking bad news: another feature of being in many of the health professions is the fact of having to tell people things they would probably rather not hear;
- breaking good news: underrated, the skill of telling people good things is also vital;
- teaching patients or clients: the accent in health care is increasingly on prevention and part of that prevention is helping people to learn how to care for themselves; teaching skills are also discussed at length in this book;
- teaching staff/colleagues: many senior health professionals also have a teaching responsibility for younger or more junior colleagues;
- speaking at meetings: most health care managers and educators become committee members and being a good one involves learning certain, basic skills;
- chairing meetings: similarly, the ability to chair a meeting involves various learning processes; unfortunately the skills of chairing meetings are rarely taught formally and many health care professionals have to pick up the skill by simply observing others at work;
- evaluating colleagues' performance: quality assurance means that all health professionals are evaluated and many have to evaluate others;
- disciplining colleagues: a form of assertive behaviour, perhaps, appropriate use of disciplinary procedures constitute a small part of many health care managers' roles.

An even more comprehensive list of possible interpersonal skills in health care is offered in Figure 3.1. It is worth reflecting on the list and seeing if you can add to it. The aim is also to show that interpersonal skills, in everyday life, do not always revolve around counselling, group facilitation, being assertive and so forth. The point of discussing skills such as counselling, though, is that they serve as ideal types. The micro-skills involved in counselling are also skills to be found in everyday, more down-to-earth exchanges between health care professionals and their clients or patients.

All health care professionals need and use a variety of interpersonal skills in every aspect of their work. The difficult thing, however, is how to teach these skills to other people. Very often, they are learned through the process known as 'sitting with Nellie': the new health care professional is supposed to pick up

Acting as an ambassador for the
organization
Admitting you were wrong
Answering the phone
Apologizing
Arguing
Attending a tribunal
Avoiding certain topics
Being a go-between
Being an advocate
Breaking bad news
Breaking up arguments
Chairing a conference
Chairing a discussion
Chairing a formal meeting
Chatting
Controlling feelings
Correcting another person
Counselling
Countering someone else's argument
Criticizing
Defending a colleague
Defending an idea
Defending an opinion
Describing
Disagreeing
Disciplining
Dissuading
Distracting
Encouraging
Expressing feelings
Giving a conference paper
Giving a presentation to colleagues
Giving a report
Giving advice
Giving an opinion
Giving information
Giving instructions
Helping
Instructing
Interrupting
Introducing self
Inviting ideas
Listening
Mediating
Negotiating
Offering a verbal assessment

Participating in a group
Passing judgement
Passing on information
Passing the time of day
Persuading
Reasoning
Receiving bad news
Receiving good news
Rectifying a mistake
Remaining silent
Returning goods
Saying 'no'
Saying 'sorry'
Saying goodbye
Saying goodbye to a group of people
Seeking opinions
Selling an idea
Sharing a joke
Sharing feelings
Sharing good news
Sharing ideas
Sharing self
Sharing thoughts
Showing appropriate anger
Speaking over an intercom system
Sticking to a point of view
Supporting
Supporting relatives
Supporting someone else's argument
Switching your viewpoint
Taking instructions
Talking on radio/television
Talking to patients
Talking to colleagues
Talking to people from other
disciplines
Talking to the press
Talking while carrying out a
procedure
Teaching patients/clients
Teaching peers
Teaching students
Thanking an individual
Thanking people in a group
Using the telephone
Welcoming guests

Figure 3.1 A more comprehensive list of interpersonal skills in the health care
professions

various skills through observing older and more experienced colleagues at
work. The second problem arises when those colleagues demonstrate that they
do not have particular interpersonal skills! Arguably, again, this situation has

arisen because those colleagues were also given no formal training and so the cycle of events is complete. This chapter sets out to explore how interpersonal skills may be taught to health care professionals.

OVERSIMPLIFICATION: A WARNING

While this book is about practical and fairly straightforward ways of helping people to develop and enhance their interpersonal skills, a note of caution should also be sounded. Personal relationships – of any sort – are complicated and we should not understimate that complexity. Quite apart from people's behaviours and feelings in relationships, we have, 'sitting behind' those things, people's motives and intentions. These are much less visible and much more difficult to study or penetrate. Consider, for example, the potential variables that **may** lay behind the initial meeting of a nurse with her new patient.

The **nurse** may be:

- trying to create a good impression of the organization;
- trying to create a good impression of herself;
- attracted to the patient;
- repelled by the patient;
- trying to hide her feelings;
- trying to create the impression that she is busy;
- trying to hide the fact that she is busy;
- reminded, by the patient, of someone else she knows and likes;
- reminded, by the patient, of someone else she knows and dislikes;
- trying to work as quickly as possible;
- embarrassed;
- flustered

and so on.
The **patient** may be:

- trying to act the 'good patient';
- genuinely happy to please;
- attracted to the nurse;
- not wanting to take up more time than necessary;
- wanting the nurse's full attention;
- wanting to be reassured;
- annoyed by the nurse;
- upset by 'the system';
- disturbed by his illness;
- worried about conditions at home;
- worried about relatives;
- embarrassed;

- happy to be in hospital;
- frightened of hospitals and wanting people to know;
- frightened of hospitals and trying to hide the fact;
- depressed

and so on.

Both may be:

- interested in forming a relationship;
- not interested in forming a relationship;
- ready to help each other;
- antagonistic towards one another

and so on.

In either case, each person may only glimpse the intentions or motives of the other. They may not even glimpse them at all. Certainly there is more going on 'beneath the surface' in any exchange and in any relationship and we would do well to remain modest about the degree to which we really can 'know' other people with whom we come in contact.

The situation is further complicated by the fact that the 'actor' – the person displaying a certain behaviour may or may not be aware of all of his intentions or motives. We do not have to enter into a debate about the Freudian notion of the unconscious mind to appreciate that sometimes we are aware of why we are doing something, as we do it and sometimes we only become aware of why we are doing something after the event. Sometimes, too, we only appreciate our own intentions and motives after another person has offered a view on our behaviour. At least two possibilities exist here. First is the possibility that this *post hoc* description of our intentions and motives really does match the intentions and motives that we had at the time of acting. The other possibility is that we chose to adopt the idea of those intentions and motives, after the event, because we 'like' the explanation. In the end, there is no foolproof way of knowing what our 'real' intentions are at any given time and even fewer ways of knowing what other peoples' real intentions are. The popular view is sometimes that we can glimpse other people's motives through their 'body language' – through the sometimes apparent contradiction, between what people are saying and what their bodies are doing. However, this method of analysis is far from foolproof. A simple example will serve here.

It is sometimes felt that folded arms are a sign of 'defensiveness' and that the person who talks while folding his or her arms is somehow less 'open' than the person who does not do this. However, a moment's reflection will reveal that there are plenty of other possible explanations for why a person might do this. These might include the fact that the person was cold, that he was in the habit of folding his arms, that he had **no** particular 'reason' for crossing his arms, to name but a few. This whole issue highlights the eternal problem of understanding other people's minds. There **is** no known way of achieving this sort of understanding: all our theories about why people do what they do and how they do it are just that: theories. We would do well to bear this in mind when tempted to 'interpret' the behaviour of others or to best-guess their motives or intentions. I am reminded here of the dictum of George Kelly, the personal construct theorist who suggested that 'if you want to know what someone is about, **ask** them, they might just tell you.' And we might add: 'and, as a rule, **believe them**, when they do'. Banyard and Hayes (1994) offer a useful comment on these issues:

> The topic of non-verbal communication is a great favourite with popularizers of psychology. Observing standing, sitting or walking styles and deciding what each might mean has an obvious appeal – whether it is based on reality or not. It is the psychology of magazine articles, which address non-verbal communication in times such as 'If you cross your legs when talking to your boss it means ...' or 'If you put your weight on your left foot when standing at a bus stop it means ...'. This type of analysis, understandably, is of very little value indeed – it is too simplistic to take account of the real subtleties involved in human communication and only the very credulous follow its blueprints.

The other point to bear in mind is that all behaviour is contextual. What something 'means' in one context may not mean the same thing in another. How one person acts in one situation is no guarantee or how he or she might act in another. We all act out certain roles – professional and personal. We are all engaged, too, in complex games of trying to assess what effect our behaviour will have on others. Others are also trying to assess how their behaviour will affect us. Finally, we attach all sorts of attributions to other people. We infer things from the way they dress, from the things that they do and from the things that they say – regardless of whether or not these attributions really are the case. Pennington summarizes three important facets of attribution theory as follows:

- We constantly try to explain our own behaviour and that of other people. This process helps to reduce uncertainty as we attribute causes.
- We are constantly searching for and using information as we attribute causes.
- We are like naive scientists because we are continually engaged in the business of trying to describe, explain and predict social behaviour (Pennington, 1986).

In this way, we skirt around each other, sometimes being 'honest' with ourselves and others and sometimes being less so. Sometimes, it is possible to catch ourselves acting in this sort of way. At other times, we are oblivious even to our own game playing. Such, then, are some of the complications of trying to make sense of interpersonal behaviour.

One constant in the range of research projects that have been carried out into what is viewed at interpersonally 'effective' behaviour is the fact that personal qualities seem to be important. Skills, it would seem, are useful, but what people look for when they are deciding whether or not to talk to us about their problems is whether or not they feel we have the appropriate personal attributes. In a study in which we asked the question 'what does an interpersonally skilled person "look like"' of a wide range of health care workers – using Kelly's repertory grid method – we found, time and time again, that it was not skills that were identified but the personal qualities of others that were described as important 'ingredients' of an interpersonally skilled person (Burnard and Morrison, 1989). An added layer of complexity, in this field, is that what makes up any single person's list of what contributes 'ideal' personal qualities seems likely to differ from another person's list. What I look for in another person may be different to what you look for. Despite this, and with caution, we can make a few hesitant generalizations.

The subtle aspects of interpersonal skills

Despite the reservations, above, it remains true, I think, that communication takes place between people on a subtle level as well as on a concrete, overt level. Much of the meaning of an interaction is bound up in looks, gestures, slight changes in facial expressions, shared meanings and so on. Interpersonal skills are by no means easily reduced to simple and clear-cut skills. The novelist Harold Brodkey catches this 'subtle' level of comunication in his wonderfully over-qualified sentence in *Profane Friendship* (Brodkey, 1995). He is describing the slow development of a relationship between two people and writes:

> The possibility of liking each other was slightly apparent in this tone and that look.

I am never sure how to describe these subtle aspects. Some people like to use the term 'intuition' to summarize this 'unstatable' aspect but the word seems to have been so overused as to be meaningless. It does seem clear, though, that we communicate on a wide range (and depth) of levels and the best we can do, perhaps, is to 'remain awake' and to continue to be ready for the more subtle signals as they appear.

PERSONAL QUALITIES

Prior to any discussion about the skills themselves comes an appreciation of certain personal qualities that are a necessary prerequisite of effective interpersonal relationship. A basic cluster of such necessary qualities may be identified as: warmth and genuineness, empathy, and unconditional positive regard (Rogers, 1967). These personal qualities cannot accurately be described as 'skills' but they are necessary if we are to use interpersonal skills effectively and caringly. They form the basis and the bedrock of all effective human relationships.

ACQUIRING INTERPERSONAL SKILLS IN THE HEALTH PROFESSIONS: NUMBER 7

Using 'trigger' films for discussion

Select pieces of films or prepare your own, that illustrate a small bit of interpersonal behaviour. The clip should not be more than three or four minutes long. Use the clip or a series of them to trigger off discussion in an interpersonal skills training course.

Warmth and genuineness

Warmth, in the health care relationship refers to an ability to be approachable and open to the another person. Schulman (1982) argues that the following characteristics are involved in demonstrating the concept of warmth: equal worth, absence of blame, non-defensiveness and closeness. Warmth is as much a frame of mind as a skill and perhaps one developed through being honest with yourself and being prepared to be open with others. It also involves treating the other person as an equal human being. Martin Buber (1958) discusses the difference between the 'I–it' relationship and the 'I–Thou (or 'I–you') relationship. In the I–it relationship, one person treats the other as an object, as a thing. In the I–thou relationship, there occurs a meeting of persons, transcending any differences there may be in terms of status, background, lifestyle, belief or value systems. In the I–thou relationship there is a sense of sharing and of mutuality, a sense that can be contagious and is of particular value in the health care relationship. Meyeroff describes this well in his classic book on caring:

> In a meaningful friendship, caring is mutual, each cares for the other: caring becomes contagious. My caring for the other helps activate his caring for me; and similarly his caring for me helps activate my caring for him, it 'strengthens' me to care for him (Meyeroff, 1972).

What is not clear is the degree to which a health care relationship can be a mutual relationship. Rogers (1967) argues that the health care relationship can be a mutual relationship but Buber acknowledges that because it is always the client who seeks out the health care professional and comes to that health care professional with problems, the relationship is, necessarily, unequal and lacking in mutuality. For Buber, the professional relationship starts and progresses from an unequal footing:

> He comes for help to you. You don't come for help to him. And not only this, but you are able, more or less to help him. He can do different things to you, but not help you ... You are, of course, a very important person for him. But not a person whom he wants to see and to know and is able to.

He is floundering around, he comes to you. He is, may I say, entangled in your life, in your thoughts, in your being, your communication, and so on. But he is not interested in you as you. It cannot be (Buber, 1966).

Thus warmth must be offered by the health care professional but the feeling may not necessarily be reciprocated by the client. There is, as well, another problem with the notion of warmth. We all perceive personal qualities in different sorts of ways. One person's warmth is another person's sickliness or sentimentality. We cannot guarantee how our 'warmth' will be perceived by the other person. In a more general way, however, 'warmth' may be compared to 'coldness'. It is clear that the 'cold' person would not be the ideal person to undertake helping another person in a health care setting! It is salutary, however, to reflect on the degree to which there are 'cold' people working in the health care arena and to question why this may be so. It is possible that interpersonal skills training may help this situation for it may be that some 'cold' people are unaware of their coldness.

On the other hand, we might not want to argue that only 'warm people' are interpersonally effective. It seems likely that different people respond to different qualities in others. Some, it seems likely, are going to want to talk to someone who is detached and unemotional. The idea that everyone has to be warm in order to be good at helping others seems to be something of an exaggeration.

To a degree, however, our relationships with others tend to be self-monitoring. To a degree, we anticipate, as we go on with a relationship, the effect we are having on others and modify our presentation of self accordingly. Thus we soon get to know if our 'warmth' is too much for the client or is being perceived by him in a negative way. This ability to monitor ourselves and our relationships constantly is an important part of the process of developing interpersonal skills.

Genuineness, too, is another important aspect of the relationship. In one sense, the issue is black or white. We either genuinely care for the person in front of us or we do not. We cannot easily fake professional interest. We must be interested. Some people, however, will interest us more than others. Often, those clients who remind us of our own problems or our own personalities will interest us most of all. This is not so important as our having a genuine interest in the fact that the relationship is happening at all.

On the surface of it, there may appear to be a conflict between the concept of genuineness and the self-monitoring alluded to, above. Self-monitoring may be thought of as 'artificial' or contrived and therefore not genuine. The 'genuineness', discussed here, relates to the health care professional's interest in the human relationship that is developing between the two people. Any ways in which that relationship can be enhanced must serve a valuable purpose. It is quite possible to be 'genuine' and yet aware of what is happening: genuine and yet committed to increasing interpersonal competence.

There is, though, an interesting paradox contained within the idea of being a 'genuine' professional. If we are open to the idea of learning interpersonal skills, then it is hard to argue, at the same time, that these 'learned skills' are genuine – at least, initially. Almost by definition, the person who is learning a range of new skills is not genuine. At least, not in their actions. They may, perhaps, be genuine in the intention to help and this may help us to understand this approach to 'being genuine'. Perhaps, too, after a while, the acquired skills become part of the make up of the person and become genuine through continual use.

A summing-up of the notion of genuineness in the context of helping the health care professions was provided by Egan when he identified the following aspects of it:

You are genuine in your relationship with your clients when you:

- do not overemphasise your professional role and avoid stereotyped role behaviours;
- are spontaneous but not uncontrolled or haphazard in your relationships;
- remain open and non-defensive even when you feel threatened;
- are consistent and avoid discrepancies – between your values and your behaviour, and between your thoughts and your words in interactions with clients – while remaining respectful and reasonably tactful;
- are willing to share yourself and your experience with clients if it seems helpful (Egan, 1986).

There is another sense of genuineness and that lies in the notion of being 'ordinary'. In this sense, 'genuine' means 'being yourself' and avoiding the putting on of a professional front. We must be as we really are. This concept is well demonstrated in the following extract of a discussion between a therapist and his client. In it, the client, for a moment, glimpses the 'humanness' of the therapist:

One woman said 'I had a bad weekend. Other people are stable. I'm so up and down. I hide my rockiness'. I said, 'Don't we all'. She: 'You too?' I: 'Does that surprise you?' She: 'Well I guess not. You're human too.' I understood that to mean she also felt human, at least for the moment (Basescu, 1990).

The idea of remaining ordinary and 'like other people' is captured, too, by the interviewer and monologuist, Spalding Gray, when he describes part of an interview that he carried out, in front of an audience, in a New England town.

I asked if she had any last questions, and she said, 'Yes. When are you going to get a hairpiece?' I was thrown by that one. 'What, do you really think I need one?' She said 'Well, you're a world-renowned talk-show host. I don't know how you can do talk shows with that bald spot.' (Gray, 1985)

If anyone has the capacity to 'stay ordinary' in a range of ordinary and extra-ordinary situations, Spalding Gray has, and his books are well worth reading as examples of the 'ordinary inside the extraordinary'.

Learning warmth and genuineness

Can a person learn to be warm and genuine? It is arguable that we have learned all our personal qualities so why should we imagine that a person is somehow 'naturally' warm and genuine or not as the case may be? Clearly these qualities cannot be learned in the same way as skills. They can, however, be developed through the person's awareness of them as qualities at all and through that person striving to pay attention to the other person, to forego artifice and the adoption of a 'professional veneer'. If we are truly to help others, we cannot do so if we are trying to maintain a particular posture or trying too hard to be professional. We must, instead, come to the client as we are. We must learn to be ourselves.

Empathic understanding

Empathy is a relatively new term, apparently coined by Titchner in 1909 to translate the German term *'Einfuhlung'* (Bateson and Coke, 1981). The term is usually used to convey the idea of the ability to enter the perceptual world of the other person: to see the world as they see it. It also suggests an ability to convey this perception to the other person. Kalisch (1971) defines empathy as 'the ability to perceive accurately the feelings of another person and to communicate this understanding to him'. Meyeroff describes empathic understanding from the point of view of caring for another person:

> To care for another person I must be able to understand him and his world as if I were inside it. I must be able to see, as it were, with his eyes what his world is like to him and how he sees himself. Instead of merely looking at him in a detached way from outside, as if he were a specimen I must be able to be with him in his world, 'going' into his world in order to sense from 'inside' what life is like for him, what he is striving to be, and what he requires to grow (Meyeroff, 1972).

Empathy is different to sympathy. Sympathy suggests 'feeling sorry' for the other person or, perhaps, identifying with how they feel. If a person sympathizes they imagine themselves as being in the other person's position. With empathy the person tries to imagine how it is to be the other person. Feeling sorry for that person does not really come into it. On the other hand, the two concepts of sympathy and empathy are not always that easy to separate. Will Self suggests the following in his novel *My Idea of Fun*:

What do you think that the definition of 'empathy' is? Jot it down on a scrap of paper if it helps you to fix it in your mind. Now go and look these two definitions up in the dictionary. I think you'll find that you've got them the wrong way round, that what you thought was empathy is really sympathy and vice versa. You see, that's been my problem – all the time I thought I was sympathising I was really empathising. I'm not going to make big claims about this semantic quirk but I do think it's worth remarking on, for when two key terms bumble over one another in this fashion you can be sure that something is afoot (Self, 1994).

Perhaps sympathy and empathy are closer that we sometimes imagine. Indeed, dictionary definitions often **do** confirm Self's point.

The process of developing empathy involves something of an act of faith. When we empathize with another person, we cannot know what the outcome of that empathizing will be. If we pre-empt the outcome of our empathizing, we are already not empathizing – we are thinking of solutions and of ways of influencing the client towards a particular goal that we have in mind.

Hough (1994) describes empathy as follows:

The word 'empathy' is used to describe a particular characteristic which the counsellor should possess in relation to the client. When a counsellor is empathic it means that she is capable of understanding the client in the very deepest sense, that she can, when necessary, stand in the client's shoes and perceive things as the client perceives them, and that she can also transmit this deep understanding back to the client who will be encouraged and supported by it. This ability to enter the true spirit or feelings of another person's world is sometimes referred to as being within the client's 'frame of reference'. It is quite different to sympathy because sympathy is concerned with feelings of pity, compassion or tenderness towards another person, whereas empathy requires much more effort, concentration and discipline.

The process of empathizing involves entering into the perceptual world of the other person without, necessarily knowing where that process will lead to. Martin Buber, mystic and writer on psychotherapy, summed up well this mixture of willingness to explore the world of the other without presupposing the outcome, when he wrote the following metaphor:

A man lost his way in a great forest. After awhile another lost his way and chanced on the first. Without knowing what had happened to him, he asked the way out of the woods.

'I don't know', said the first. 'But I can point out the ways that lead further into the thicket, and after that let us try to find the way together'.
(Buber, 1948)

Developing empathic understanding is the process of exploring the client's world, with the client, neither judging nor necessarily offering advice. Perhaps it can be achieved best through the process of carefully attending and listening to the other person and, perhaps, by use of the skill known as 'reflection' that is discussed elsewhere in this book. It is also a 'way of being', a disposition towards the client, a willingness to explore the other person's problems and to allow the other person to express themselves fully. Again, as with all aspects of the 'client-centred' approach to caring, the empathic approach is underpinned by the idea that it is the client, in the end, who will find their own way through and will find their own answers to their problems in living. To be empathic is to be a fellow traveller, a friend to the person as they undertake the search. Empathic understanding, then, invokes the notion of 'befriending'.

There are, of course, limitations to the degree to which we can truly empathize. Because we all live in different 'worlds' based on our particular culture, education, physiology, belief systems and so forth, we all view that world slightly differently. Thus, to truly empathize with another person would involve actually becoming that other person! We can, however, strive to get as close to the perceptual world of the other by listening and attending and by suspending judgement. We can also learn to forget ourselves, temporarily and give ourselves as completely as we can to the other person. There is an interesting paradox involved here. First, we need self-awareness to enable us to develop empathy. Then we need to forget ourselves in order to truly give our empathic attention to the other person.

Learning empathy

Empathy can be developed through the use of experiential learning methods. Emphasizing, as they do, listening, the sharing of experience and a pluralistic view of the world, such exercises soon encourage group participants to pay attention to what someone else is saying and to resist the temptation always to compare my experience with your experience.

The simple listening exercises offered in the final chapter of this book are a good starting place for learning empathy. Beyond these excercises, too, is the need to develop consciously the ability to put ourselves into the frame of reference of the other person. As we have seen, to some degree this means forgetting ourselves, our belief and value systems and suspending judgement on what we hear. Our aim is not to criticize or to judge but to listen and understand what the other person is trying to convey.

Unconditional positive regard

Carl Rogers's phrase 'unconditional positive regard' (Rogers, 1967) conveys a particularly important predisposition towards the client, by the health care professional. Rogers also called it 'prizing' or even just 'accepting'. It means that the client is viewed with dignity and valued as a worthwhile and positive human being. The 'unconditional' prefix refers to the idea that such regard is offered without any preconditions. Often in relationships, some sort of reciprocity is demanded: I will like you (or love you) as long as you return that liking or loving. Rogers is asking that the feelings that the health care professional holds for the client should be undemanding and not requiring reciprocation. There is a suggestion of an inherent 'goodness' within the client, bound up in Rogers's notion of unconditional positive regard. This notion of people as essentially good can be traced back, at least, to Rousseau's *Emile* and is philosophically problematic. Arguably, notions such as 'goodness' and 'badness' are social constructions and to argue that a person is born good or bad is fraught. However, as a practical starting point in the health care relationship, it seems to be a good idea that we assume an inherent, positive and life-asserting characteristic in the client. It seems difficult to argue otherwise. It would be odd, for instance, to engage in the process of helping another person with the view that the person was essentially bad, negative and unlikely to grow or develop! Thus, unconditional positive regard offers a baseline from which to start the health care relationship. In order to grasp this concept further, it will be useful to refer directly to Roger's definition of the notion as it relates to the counselling, therapy and the health care setting:

> I hypothesize that growth and change are more likely to occur the more that the counsellor is experiencing a warm, positive, accceptant attitude towards what is the client. It means that he prizes his client, as a person, with the same quality of feeling that a parent feels for his child, prizing him as a person regardless of his particular behaviour at the moment. It means that he cares for his client in a non-possessive way, as a person with potentialities. It involves an open willingness for the client to be whatever feelings are real in him at the moment – hostility or tenderness, rebellion or submissiveness, assurance or self-depreciation. It means a kind of love for the client as he is, providing we understand the word love as equivalent to the theologian's term agape, and not in its usual romantic and possessive meanings. What I am describing is a feeling which is not paternalistic, nor sentimental, nor superficially social and agreeable. It respects the other person as a separate individual and does not possess him. It is a kind of liking which has strength, and which is not demanding. We have termed it positive regard (Rogers and Stevens, 1967).

Unconditional positive regard, then, involves a deep and positive feeling for the other person, perhaps equivalent, in the health professions to what Alistair Campbell has called 'moderated love' (Campbell, 1984). He talks of 'lovers and professors', suggesting that certain professionals profess to love, thus claiming both the ability to be professional and to express altruistic love or disinterested love for others. It is interesting that Campbell seems to be suggesting that a health care professional can 'professionally care' or even 'professionally love' her client. The suggestion is also that the health profession has a positive and warm confidence in her own skills and abilities in the health care relationship. Such an outlook is also supported by Egan who, in his 'portrait of a helper' says:

> They respect their clients and express this respect by being available to them, working with them, not judging them, trusting the constructive forces found in them, and ultimately placing the expectation on them that they will do whatever is necessary to handle their problems in living more effectively (Egan, 1990).

I suspect, though, that, in the end, Rogers is asking too much of therapists and others to offer unconditional positive regard. While we might feel it for some people, it seems unlikely that we will experience it with everyone of our clients or patients. And yet that does not need to mean that we cannot be helpful to them. I suspect that we can, sometimes, have a 'businesslike' approach to some clients and still help them. Nor, I suspect, does every client want us to experience or express unconditional positive regard. Some, I suspect, would like a more detached relationship. The idea that every therapeutic relationship necessarily has to be a close and accepting one does not, in my experience, seem borne out in clinical practice.

Learning unconditional positive regard

Learning not to judge others often comes through accepting ourselves. We judge others more harshly when we have not resolved various personal problems. We judge even more readily when we do not know what our personal problems are! It is suggested, again, that the route to learning unconditional positive regard may begin with the development of self-awareness. While we cannot hope to sort ourselves out totally, as health professionals helping other people with their problems, it seems reasonable that we begin by at least becoming aware of some of our own.

ACQUIRING INTERPERSONAL SKILLS IN THE HEALTH PROFESSIONS: NUMBER 8

Giving positive feedback

It is often quite easy to tell other people what annoys us about them. Try telling people you work with or live with how much you appreciate what they do. This can be used (often with much hilarity) in a group context. Each member of the group says what they like or appreciate about each other member, in turn.

THERAPEUTIC INTERPERSONAL SKILLS IDENTIFIED

Now it is possible to identify certain core, therapeutic interpersonal skills and offer clear descriptions of the stages of training that may be offered in workshops aimed at developing those skills. The style of training is that based on the notion of experiential learning, discussed in the last chapter. The argument is that the only way to learn interpersonal skills is to engage in them. They can be lectured upon, discussed and generally dissected but they will not be effectively learned until the learner uses them. The recurrent theme, throughout this chapter (and throughout this book), is how to offer people experiences that will help them to develop their own particular but effective style of interacting with others.

It will be noted that counselling skills are argued to be the bedrock type of interpersonal skill upon which all others are built. It is asserted that the health care professional who can learn to use a wide range of effective counselling skills is well on the way to being interpersonally competent. The fact that the person who is counselling has to deal with so many different aspects of the human condition suggests that the one who can counsel effectively is likely to be able to transfer those skills to a variety of other interpersonal situations.

COUNSELLING SKILLS

Counselling skills may be used in a variety of health care settings. They may be used to help the person who is suffering from a temporary emotional crisis or they may be helpful in caring for the person who has longer term problems in living. They may also be practical and useful as a set of interpersonal skills for everyday use in every client–practitioner situation. Counselling skills, after all, are not skills to be turned on and off according to the need but a 'way of being' with the client to enable them to communicate their thoughts and feelings more effectively. Counselling skills form the basis of all effective interpersonal relationships between the health care professional and the health care consumer, whatever the relationship between those two people. Further, the skills are essential ones for helping other colleagues. A short list of situations in which counselling skills are useful in all of the caring professions includes:

- helping relatives to cope with bereavement;
- working with children and adolescents;
- helping families to work through problems;
- discussing psychiatric difficulties and making decisions about when to 'refer on' to other health care professionals;
- helping other colleagues;
- teaching students to become counsellors.

DEFINING COUNSELLING

Counselling has been discussed considerably in the recent press and by those in the health professions. One of the things that causes problems is the diversity of definitions that exist for the term.

Noonan offered a definition that reflects an historical view to the activity but, oddly, noted too that it was a 'popular activity'.

Counselling has its beginnings, both historically as an emerging discipline and daily as a popular activity, in many different professions. It fills the gap between psychotherapy and friendship, and it has become a recognised extension of the work of almost everyone whose business touches upon the personal, social, occupational, medical, educational and spiritual aspects of people (Noonan, 1983).

Aptekar, on the other hand, saw it as a 'private activity' that did not, necessarily, need to be a professional one.

Counselling can be carried out privately, and without the need to call on agency resources ... all that is required is a person who has a problem and one who is willing to share that problem and bring to bear upon it whatever skills he may have, so that a solution may be reached (Aptekar, 1955).

Writing from the point of view of counselling children, Crompton identified a range of specific foci as a means of defining counselling.

[Counselling is] help, through the development of a professional relationship, to recognise and manage problems and difficulties connected with and/or stimulated by a range of factors including environment (for example, school), event (for example, bereavement), individual development (for example, sexual), relationship (for example, with parents), movement (for example, within care, between divorced parents), behaviour (for example, offending), and to assist with growth and development in all aspects of the individual person – cognitive, emotional, physical and spiritual (Crompton, 1992).

Meanwhile, Jones took a more obviously 'humanistic' approach to definition when defining it as a process leading to personal growth and responsibility.

An enabling process, designed to help an individual come to terms with his life and grow to greater maturity through learning to take responsibility and to make decisions for himself (Jones, 1984).

Mallon highlights the variety of forms of counselling and, from an educational point of view, defined it thus:

Counselling happens in many settings, at many times and in many different ways. It is not restricted to private rooms where a confident, fully trained counsellor receives those who wish to be helped. Rather, in most educational settings, a somewhat harried adult searched for a quiet space in which to snatch some time for a distressed child or parent to talk. The contact is often brief, unplanned and unsatisfactory for all concerned, though in many instances it is the best that is available at the time (Mallon, 1987).

Breese, noted the time factor involved in counselling.

[Counselling is] offering a chance to talk freely and openly, individually or in a group in a non-authoritarian atmosphere, on a regular (normally weekly) basis, within a structure of time and place where people have the opportunity a) to be heard and understood; b) to see things from the point of view of others; and c) to gain greater understanding of themselves and others (Breese, 1983).

Reber took a general, open and fairly versatile approach to definition and suggested that counselling involved many of the processes found in education itself.

A generic term that is used to cover the several processes of interviewing, testing, guiding, advising etc., designed to help an individual solve problems, plan for the future etc. (Reber, 1985).

Elsewhere, I have focussed a definition on the need for counselling to involve not only talking but also the need for **action**.

The process of counselling is the means by which one person helps another to clarify his or her life situation and to decide further lines of action (Burnard, 1994).

Rowe offered a slightly ironic view of counselling and suggested one way in which counselling might differ from psychotherapy.

If people feel that psychotherapy is too pretentious a word to apply to what they do, they describe what they do as counselling (Rowe in Masson, 1990).

The British Association for Counselling seemed to want to cover all possible aspects of counselling in their definition and, again, offered a broadly humanistic definition:

the skilled and principled use of a relationship to facilitate self-knowledge, emotional acceptance and growth, and the optimal development of personal resources. The overall aim is to provide the opportunity to work towards living more satisfyingly and resourcefully. Counselling ... may be concerned with development issues, addressing and resolving personal insights and knowledge, working through feelings of inner conflict or improving relationships with others (BAC, 1989a).

The approach taken by Nelson-Jones illustrated that, unsurprisingly (as a writer on the topic), he had considered a wide range of aspects of the usage of the term.

The term 'counselling' is used in a number of ways. For instance, counselling may be viewed: as a special kind of *helping relationship*; as a *repertoire of interventions*; as a *psychological process*; or in terms of its *goals*, or the *people who counsel*, or its *relationship to psychotherapy* (Nelson-Jones, 1995).

Nelson-Jones, perhaps, offers the most exhaustive of definitions and the definition with the broadest scope. It is interesting to review these definitions and to note that some of them define counselling in term of the **aims** of counselling, some in terms of what counsellors do and some attempt to summarize the features that comprise the counselling relationship. All of these definitions can be compared and contrasted with definitions of **psychotherapy** – something with which counselling is often confused:

> In the most inclusive sense [psychotherapy is] the use of absolutely any technique or procedure that has palliative or curative effects upon any mental, emotional or behavioural disorder. In this general sense the term is neutral with regard to the theory that may underlie it, the actual procedures and techniques entailed or the form and duration of the treatment. There may, however, be legal and professional issues involved in the actual practice of what is called psychotherapy, and ... the term is properly used only when it is carried out by someone with recognised training and using accepted techniques (Reber, 1985).

> [Psychotherapy is] the systematic use of a relationship between therapist and patient – as opposed to pharmacological or social methods – to produce changes in cognition, feelings or behaviour (Holmes and Lindley, 1991).

A scathing attack on therapy is made by King-Spooner (1995). In noting the lack of empirical evidence to support the efficacy (or otherwise) of psychotherapy, he compares psychotherapy to an animal that is about to become extinct:

> Psychotherapy waddles, bloated with self-congratulation, through a benign undergrowth of conferences, workshops, consulting rooms, congenial journals, its strongest characteristics if not its defining expression one of inane amiability (King-Spooner, 1995).

King-Spooner goes on to argue that psychotherapy is so ill-defined, attracts such little criticism within its own ranks and is so difficult to research that it seems to be 'held together' by practitioners and theorists who tend to agree with each other.

Woolfe, Dryden and Charles-Edwards summarize the differences that are sometimes argued to exist between the counselling and psychotherapy. They suggest that the following points are made:

(a) that psychotherapy is concerned with personality change whereas counselling is concerned with helping the individual to utilize his or her own resources;

(b) that psychotherapy is concerned with people who are in some sense 'neurotic' or psychologically disturbed, whereas counselling is concerned with people who are basically emotionally healthy but who are confronted by a temporary life problem or issue;

(c) that whereas the focus of methodology for the psychotherapist is the nature of transference between therapist and client, the counsellor is less concerned with this relationship that with helping the client to clarify the issues and develop strategies of management by the counsellor's deployment of a specific set of relatively restricted skills;

(d) that the psychotherapist is concerned with the inner world of the client as opposed to the counsellor's focus on helping the client to resolve external issues which are generating problems;

(e) that the work of the psychotherapist is based on psychoanalytical theory, whereas the counsellor's work is inspired by humanistic approaches;

(f) that psychotherapists tend to work in medical settings, whereas counsellors tend to work in non-medical environments; thus, the former work with patients and the latter with clients;

(g) that counselling tends to be a shorter-term process than psychotherapy, and vice versa (Woolfe, Dryden and Charles-Edwards, 1989).

These points are problematic. It may be difficult to state exactly what the difference is between 'personality change' and 'utilizing your own resources'. Some may question the idea that psychotherapy is 'concerned with people ... who are neurotic'. Arguably, many 'normal' people also benefit (or otherwise) from psychotherapy. 'Transference' may be acknowledged in a psychodynamic approach to psychotherapy but not, necessarily, in other sorts. Presumably, too, the notion of transference would be important to a **counsellor** who practised from a psychodynamic point of view. Also, the distinction made between psychotherapy being concerned with an 'inner' world, with counselling being more externally focused seems particularly contentious. The point about psychotherapy being based on psychoanalytical theory only applies to psychotherapy that **is** psychodynamic in orientation. There are plenty of other psychotherapies that are **not** psychodynamic. Finally, the idea that psychotherapists tend to work in medical settings while counsellors tend to work in 'non-medical environments' is not born out by exploring directories of therapists and counsellors. There are many 'medical' counsellors working in hospitals and GP practices and many 'non-medical' therapists working in the community at large.

As can be seen, the problem is by no means a simple one: there **is** a considerable amount of overlap between counselling and psychotherapy. Perhaps the most useful way of closing the debate is to view psychotherapy and counselling as two ends of a dimension, with considerable overlap between the two as illustrated in Figure 3.2.

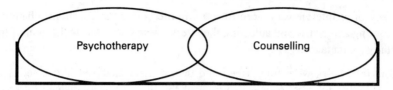

Figure 3.2 The psychotherapy and counselling dimension

HEALTH PROFESSIONALS AND COUNSELLING

To explore further the issues of counselling and psychotherapy as aspects of interpersonal skills in the health care professions, I sought the views of a small group of health professionals who fulfilled either or both of the following criteria: (a) they were trained counsellors **and** health professionals or (b) they taught counselling skills **to** health professionals.

Six health professionals who fulfilled one or both of the above criteria were invited to take part in in-depth interviews with the writer. The sample was a purposive one (May, 1993). Purposive sampling is a non-probability sampling method and one in which the respondents are chosen for the study according to the likelihood of their being able to talk on the topic in hand. If a researcher is exploring counselling with health care professionals then it is appropriate that 'health care professionals' become the population from which that sample is drawn.

LoBiondo-Wood and Haber (1994) confirm that sample sizes in qualitative studies tend to be small and suggest that interviewing should continue until 'data saturation' has occurred – that is, until no 'new' ideas or thoughts are identified by the respondents. Although a range of ideas and topics were covered in these interviews it is unlikely that data saturation occurred. Also, no attempt is being made to generalize these findings. In common with other small-scale qualitative studies, the aim is to illuminate and to offer ideas for discussion and further work.

Interviews were conducted using a semi-structured interview schedule. In a semi-structured interview, certain topics are always alluded to in each interview but the ordering and form of the questions does not necessarily remain the same. This approach to interviewing allows the interview to progress in a fairly spontaneous manner and allows for the interviewer to 'follow' rather than 'lead' the respondent. Sarantakos identifies the following characteristics of this approach and all of these points applied to the study reported here:

- Qualitative interviews use open questions only, that is questions without response categories.
- They are predominantly single interviews, questioning one person at a time.
- The question structure is not fixed or rigid, allowing change of question order, even the addition of new questions where necessary.

- They offer interviewers more freedom in presenting the questions, changing working and order, and adjusting the interview so that it meets the goal of the study (Sarantakos, 1993).

The interviews were transcribed and then content analysed into a series of themes. What follows is an elaboration of the findings accompanied by some commentary on the responses. The form of content analysis was that described by various qualitative researchers (Miles and Huberman, 1994; Field and Morse, 1995). The aim was to explore the data and to organize them according to emergent themes. These themes were partly dictated by the semi-structured interview schedule and partly through combing through the data and noting particular issues that were discussed by respondents. The analysis was partly achieved through use of the information management software program **askSam** (askSam Systems, 1994). I have described the **process** of this type of analysis, in more detail, elsewhere (Burnard, 1991; 1992a; 1992b).

Definition of counselling

Respondents offered various definitions of counselling. Sometimes, those defin-itions referred to the **purpose** or **application** of counselling:

I think that [counselling] is any kind of assistance in helping people to come to terms with an emotional or spiritual problem of any kind. It is not confined to mental distress or mental disorder. It can range from things like being in debt to having acute depression.

Another respondent offered much more of a 'textbook' definition and followed this up by suggesting some of the purposes of counselling.

Counselling is an activity in which one person is helping and one is receiving help and in which the emphasis of that help is on enabling the other person to find solutions to problems or to look at particular situa-tions which they would like resolved. Or to enable them to live more resourcefully. It involves the development, by the counsellor, of a range of particular skills but more importantly the adoption of a particular stance or attitude towards the person being helped and that includes the person feeling valued and able to explore the way in which he perceives himself and his world and not to feel judged by the counsellor.

Yet another hinted at a 'contract' but was not clear on this issue. However, as we shall see, some respondents did feel that counselling was contractual.

I think counselling is an activity in which two people agree to meet under certain conditions. And these conditions may be overt and negotiated and include such issues as confidentiality and expected outcomes. It is very much an interpersonal activity and the counsellor is there to help the client address and possibly resolve issues that are personal and meaningful to that individual.

One respondent referred to the need for the counsellor to remain **ordinary**. This idea of ordinariness in interpersonal relationships has been referred to elsewhere (Morrison, 1994). The argument is that other people are likely to respond to us more readily if we do not attempt to assume a 'professional' front or one that is 'artificial' in any way.

For me, it is a means of just being with another person who may need to talk over problems, job difficulties, personal dilemmas and so forth. In much the same way as you talk things over with a spouse or friend. That **ordinariness**, if you like, is important in counselling.

Another respondent discussed counselling in terms of 'helping people to help – a point that the respondent felt was echoed in the literature on the topic:

Counselling is creating an environment in which people can explore the issues – whatever they are, whether it is a particular way of looking at life, a childhood issue, perhaps – in a supportive atmosphere. One official definition is 'helping people to help themselves' and I quite like that: I think it's a good synopsis.

Counselling and psychotherapy

As we have seen from the discussion, above, there is plenty of contention about what does or does not differentiate counselling from psychotherapy. This contention was mirrored in the responses from respondents in the study.

Psychotherapy specifically applies to a clinical and mental illness as opposed to the neuroses that run through society. Psychotherapy is done by psychotherapists (as opposed to counsellors) and who can be lay therapists or qualified ones. Whereas counselling can be done by a whole range of people, from priests to professional counsellors.

I would guess that counselling would have a much more practical, every day, problem-solving slant to it – grounded in the here-and-now. Whereas psychotherapy, for me, evokes ideas to do with Freudian psychology ...

Another respondent hinted at the Freudian approach to psychotherapy without making the issue explicit.

I would see psychotherapy as exploring the person's life at a much deeper level including the development of insight based on exploration of early development, parental influences and those things **may** come into counselling. In counselling they are brought in to understand a **particular** situation rather than to understand the client him or herself.

The idea of the 'here-and-now' arose in another respondent's interview.

I perceive psychotherapy as being different in a variety of areas. Psychotherapists tend to be educated and trained within a particular school of practice. They tend to be in therapy themselves as part of their training. And they would claim to work with individuals at a greater depth. I see them working more in the 'there and then' than the 'here and now, ... The term is bound up with certain political issues – such as it is seen as more complex and goes on for longer and entails perhaps greater exploration and commitment on the part of the client.

One respondent had personal experience of **both** counselling and psychotherapy and made few distinctions between them. This may be a particularly important contribution to the debate given that it comes from someone who has had first-hand experience of both sorts of 'therapy'.

I've had both psychotherapy and counselling as part of my on-going training. I can't say there seems to be that much difference. Some see psychotherapy as synonymous with psychoanalysis but I find it difficult to make that distinction. Counselling doesn't go as deep as psychotherapy. Psychotherapy is a bit of a status thing as well. But there are other sorts of psychotherapy – TA [transactional analysis] and so on. I don't know really, the distinctions are blurred.

What the 'status thing' was is not made clear in the interview and was not pursued by the interviewer. The respondent **seems** to be hinting at the idea that having psychotherapy may be viewed as engaging in a 'higher status' activity than would be the case with having counselling.

Counselling and other sorts of conversation

If there were conflicting reports about what counselling and psychotherapy were, then it seemed reasonable to try to define the boundaries of counselling in another way. To this end, respondents were asked what the differences were between counselling and **other** sorts of conversation. If counselling is a discrete activity (as opposed to, for example, simply talking things over with a friend), then it seems reasonable that those who do it should be able to distinguish between simply 'talking' about something and 'doing counselling'. One respondent saw the difference in terms of **structure** – the counselling relationship was a more structured one that the more informal conversation:

The only difference that I can see is in their formal structure. If things can be achieved by talking to your friends in the pub then that's fine. Whereas counselling usually has some sort of formal structure involved. It is also a professional relationship in the sense of a counsellor and client where the counsellor is paid to counsel or listen.

It should be noted that that respondent viewed counselling as an activity that was paid for by the client. Other respondents described the differences in terms of the **roles** played out by the participants in counselling:

In counselling you would expect that one of the people has a problem, a dilemma that they are facing and that tends to be the focus of the interaction. Whereas the other person is seen as a counsellor, helper or listener. In a normal conversation that state of affairs might apply but it might also not apply and there may just be small talk about any aspect of the person's life. If you build on that definitional difference the more professional the counsellor, or the more formalized the counselling, the greater the difference would be between the helper and the helpee in terms of power, status and so forth. For example, if I go along to a friend of mine and talk about work or home problems, I won't feel guarded about status or power or being exposed psychologically because in that relationship it is guided by the principles of friendship or collegial relationships. On the other hand, if I found that I had to attend a marriage guidance counsellor, for example, I would find that rather uncomfortable. At least to begin with. And I would be very aware that I was the one with the problem and that he or she would be the person with the fix-it solution.

One is in the allocation of roles. That is the roles of helper and helpee. I think the specific aims of the conversation are to help. It is purposeful and directed towards helping and a counsellor has no other motives other than to help. People have argued that one of the differences is that the more therapeutic a conversation it is, the more likely it is to acknowledge what is happening in the here and now – in this relationship. It will include an emphasis on recognising feelings as well as thoughts. This is not to imply that ordinary conversation can't be altruistic. Egan's language of saying "helping" and of what he calls "helping" and we would call "counselling" emphasises this idea that counselling is helping. [The respondent refers to the work of Gerard Egan – see, for example, Egan, 1990.]

For another respondent, the two types of interaction were often blurred. It was sometimes difficult to say what the difference was between counselling and 'ordinary conversation'.

I think that it is a difficult question because sometimes an ordinary conversation turns into counselling and a counsellor may use counselling skills in their conversational life. I also think that counselling skills can enhance conversation and perhaps thinking as we talk about this, counselling is a specific form of conversation. I think sometimes the differences can be small and that initial sessions of clients can be 'conversational'. But they move into a counselling arena. I suspect that conversation is more reciprocal in depth and content whereas counselling tends to be less so – particularly on the part of the counsellor.

On the other hand, another respondent was **very** clear about the differences and saw them in **contractual** terms.

> Counselling has very specific parameters. There is a contract, you know how long you will meet and so on. It is a very specific type of conversation. And although some of the skills and things the counsellor may be demonstrating are similar to other conversations it is very **intentional**. It is not two-way as in other conversations. The focus in counselling is very much on the client. It is intentional focused.

What this respondent did not spell out was whether or not he felt that the contract was **implicit** rather than **explicit**. Presumably few counsellors or their clients draw up formal contracts. If, on the other hand, the contract is an implicit one, the question is raised as to whether or not the client fully understands the 'rules of the contract'.

Who does counselling?

If counselling is something to be considered as a therapeutic option by health professionals, it is important to know what sorts of people do counselling. Should they be **qualified**? Should they be 'professionals' and so on. There were various responses to this sort of question.

> Essentially anyone can do counselling. But for the most part it tends to be either professional counsellors or people who have traditionally had a counselling role, such as doctors, nurses or priests.
>
> People do counselling who are interested in other people and who are prepared to spend time with them, supporting them. Anyone could, in that respect, do counselling. Whereas in the more formal type of counselling the formal helping agencies, you get the doctors, the social workers, the lawyers, the bar tenders. Then there are the people who set themselves up as professional counsellors. I don't know people who work like that but I guess they exist.
>
> I think that counselling could be done by anyone but is more likely to be done better by someone who has had the opportunity to develop specific skills and who has been able to explore some of his characteristics and things like warmth, genuineness etc. However, it is likely that many people already possess those qualities and therefore would be better helpers than people who do not. I think there is a danger in saying that counselling is the preserve of counsellors because it relates it directly to training and I am not sure there is any evidence to demonstrate that training really does make a difference.

One respondent made a distinction between those who do counselling as part of another professional role and those who do it as a full-time job.

I would argue that there is a range of professionals whose primary professional role is working with people such as teaching, social work, nursing, medicine and in which the aim is to help others and where often that help is given through the medium of some sort of personal interaction. The more that interaction is the sole means of helping then the more we move towards that situation being counselling. For example, in medicine we see the prescribing of treatment and the relationship is not the sole means of helping. Clearly, there are some whose role is only seen as counselling and who have no other agenda. They do not have an educational agenda, a teaching agenda – the work they do is whatever the client brings. We can say then that they have a 'pure' counselling role.

Another respondent added a little to the confusion of the issues by offering a tautological response to the question of 'who counsels?' The same respondent, however, also indicates – at least, laterally, that many people could do counselling – those who were considered 'wise' and those, presumably, who had sufficient and appropriate life experience.

Counsellors do counselling! Counsellors also teach other people counselling skills in the belief that it enhances communication. I think perhaps counselling can be an unrecognised ability of those who are considered wise and of whom there aren't enough.

Most of the above respondents took the 'anyone can do counselling' approach. Others, however, wanted counselling to be more formalized and for counsellors to be trained.

People who [do counselling] are qualified counsellors. Although there may be people who have not done a proper certificate or diploma but who do counsel from experience. There are elements of counselling and counselling skills that occur in a lot of caring conversations that are carried out by health care professionals. It would be wrong to 'counsel' somebody without their permission and without a contract because of counselling's potential power.

How counselling can be used

If counselling is a therapeutic activity, it seems important to know what sorts of things counselling can be used for. These respondents were drawn from a number of sources within the transcripts.

There are a whole range of practical difficulties that can be helped by counselling, such as difficulty with study skills and getting into higher education, through to things like depression following bereavement, or neuroses or mental illnesses. There has been an expansion in the profession of counselling in recent years – you often get the situation where someone calls themselves a professional counsellor on the basis of a range of qualifications which carry no guarantee as to the likely effectiveness of that counselling. At the same time, people with a lot of experience – such as psychiatric nurses – would not, necessarily, have that qualification recognised as appropriate in counselling. I think there is a process of excluding people from counselling as an occupation going on, which is similar to the way in which health professionals exclude other people from working in health care – so that health care adopted a professional strategy for excluding people and counselling is doing the same. Counselling is becoming a work-place strategy which has the interest of the counsellor at heart and not necessarily those of the clients. The role of the qualification in counselling is exclusion rather than testing professional competence. You could have a very competent counsellor who is competent on the basis of their qualities but that would allow any number of people to become counsellors which would disrupt the professional aspirations of a lot of counsellors.

One respondent discussed the use of counselling in terms of its **structure** and how little or much the counselling relationship needed to be structured.

It can be used on a daily basis or on an informal basis with contacts with colleagues and people you are attached to. I guess this is the more informal type of counselling. Then there are the more professional settings – tutors to students for example, when you have to make yourself approachable to the students. That needs a little bit more thought. Some of the people who are tutors are therefore academic tutoring, others are there for all aspects of the student's life. Perhaps a middle path is necessary here: where tutors are prepared to listen to what is going on outside the student's immediate academic arena.

Another talked of 'formalized' counselling (as opposed, presumably, to informal or 'friendly' counselling). He noted, too, some possible **arenas** for counselling.

There is the more highly formalised counselling situation – counselling people, getting paid to do it, perhaps being part of a team helping GPs, psychiatrists etc. You may be a practitioner in a psychiatric unit or other care setting. All of these different situations are ones in which some form of counselling might be called for.

Another respondent made this distinction between 'formal' and 'informal' approaches to counselling more explicit:

There are at least two types of counselling: the informal, ordinary, unspectacular way of helping and the more professional side of things. I find that the phoniness you meet sometimes – the tilted head, the voice changing, may be a result of the training. I find that off-putting. What I need when I discuss something with somebody else is a gut reaction – a more spontaneous reaction. I would not approach a stranger for that. I would need to know the person was genuinely interested in me.

Yet another respondent talked of the difficulty of training counsellors and of the paradox between 'being spontaneous' and 'being a professional':

The spontaneous part of counselling is very very difficult to train at all. It has to do with people knowing their limitations and their likes and dislikes. As you professionalise something there is the tendency to make things more special, more detached from the real side of a relationship. Something gets lost. There is a risk of losing the spontaneous side of the interaction.

Others saw the value of counselling as laying within the process of helping people to become more responsible for themselves and re-exercising some control over what happens to them:

It can be used to enable people to examine specific problems or life situations which they would like resolved or changed. To enable them to make the best use of resources, to examine relationships, to make choices, to discover the choices available to them. To help them become more responsible for themselves and to use that responsibility over their own lives. To enable them to feel more in control of their situation. To enable them to be in a relationship with a counsellor which will enable them to develop learnings about themselves. And to make those discoveries in a situation which, although it may be uncomfortable, is safe.

It can be used to enable people to problem-solve, to identify sources of discomfort or stress and it can be used to alleviate problems of living – everyday problems of living such as anxiety and general feelings that people have of being 'outside'. It can also enhance basic communication. I can also be used, perhaps, inappropriately. It can be used as a disguise for basic disciplinary measures and it can be highjacked to disguise commercial activities such as beauty counsellors, financial counsellors etc.

Some respondents felt there was a tension between health professionals offering counselling and counselling being viewed as a 'treatment'. It was seen as essential that becoming involved in counselling should be a voluntary activity on the part of the patient or client.

I don't think there is ever a 'should' – 'this person should see a counsellor'. If they are not ready and they don't want it, then there is no point. I very much believe in people's rights to live their own life the way they want and not have counselling. When somebody is going through a traumatic experience then there are all sorts of problems that are unresolved particularly when they do not have other people in their lives to talk to.

Even when people do have lots of other people counselling is quite different. Family and friends will not talk to you in the same way. Counsellors are impartial and will not necessarily just go with you. Friends will not want to upset you whereas counselling can be more penetrating and challenging – which friends will not always be – unless they are special friends. Any sorts of problems – mid-life crises 'what's it all about' – those sorts of issues can be addressed in counselling.

When counselling should not be used

Respondents talked about when counselling **should not** be used – contraindications of counselling. These were wide ranging and are reported below. The first seems to relate to the misuse of certain sorts of training procedures.

> It shouldn't be used as a habit or for recreational purposes. I have seen some people who seem to be addicted to it. It becomes a substitution for normal human intercourse and sometimes peoples' motives are poor for going into it in the first place – such as group counselling as a place to pick up women.
>
> There may be a danger that a vulnerable person could be exposed psychologically or abused – using the term broadly. If you were, for example, attracted to a person of the opposite sex, or the same sex, that may infect the situation if you had a lot of contact with them. As a counsellor you need to be pretty solid, you need to know what you are doing and your integrity is not going to be called into question. You have to be seen as being detached but that's not a word that rests easy, you have to be comfortable in your own skin – whatever people say to you, you're not going to be tempted to abuse the relationship. Those things relate more to the professional dimension than to the ordinary side.

Sometimes, the issue was an ideological one. It was noted by one respondent that the prevailing philosophy in counselling is the 'client-centred' one in which the client is always encouraged to find his or her own solutions to his or her problems and in which direct, prescriptive intervention on the part of the counsellor is usually eschewed.

> It may depend on the type of counselling the counsellor wishes to adopt. To adopt a non-directive approach with people where it is patently obvious that you should be making suggestions, is very wasteful, I think there are lots of people who seek out help who want a direction and to keep throwing back on them and ask them to make every decision is sometimes inappropriate. People are pretty good at problem-solving and are likely to respond much better to the non-directive approach but there are people who find it difficult to make any decisions and then it is appropriate to make more concrete suggestions as to what they may do.

Sometimes, the fact that counselling was not a panacea was noted and it was made clear that counselling had very definite limitations. The following respondents highlight the problems of the then current practice of counsellors being 'to hand' after a major disaster.

There may be situations where the problem cannot be solved in your head – and I'm thinking about lack of money, serious illness, unemployment – those sorts of things. Counselling may help but some of those very serious problems aren't ones that can be solved. On these emergency situations that we see on the TV – kids drowning, accidents and things – its amazing how quickly counselling services are set up. And yet what most normal people would be is in a state of shock at that time, and its seems likely that only afterwards people need counselling – not immediately afterwards. I can't see how anyone can sit in an aircraft hangar and have twenty counsellors dashing towards them. You have the same sort of situation when children have been murdered or have disappeared and you have loads of counsellors dashing round to the school to these thirteen or fourteen year olds to do counselling, when all they need probably is to be reassured by their parents.

I think I would also disagree with those who feel that the presence of counsellors at disasters is probably inappropriate. You get a vision of 'therapeutic vultures' perhaps when people are in a extreme distress they need time to be distressed. Because counselling is not a universal panacea for the human condition.

Sometimes, the client-centred approach, referred to above, was seen as limited and one respondent called for a much wider approach to be used.

When the counsellor has other motives other than to help the client: when the counsellor is in a situation which he himself ought to take responsibility for the situation, either because of former responsibilities for it or when not to do so would cause undue pain to the client – such as when you get situations in which people steadfastly avoid giving advice by trying to be Rogerian – when the best thing would be to tell the person what to do. I recognise that in counselling you would tend to avoid that but sometimes it would be more appropriate. I think John Heron's material on prescriptive and informative interventions are quite helpful in that way.

Heron's six category intervention analysis is discussed elsewhere in this book. The question of the counsellor's 'detachment' was another issue that was discussed by some of the respondents. The issue of 'boundaries' was also discussed.

I think that where there is another relationship in which it is impossible for the counsellor to be detached – as opposed relatives, that sort of thing.

That is not to imply you can never help people close to you because I think you can. It's just that there's a way of being in counselling which is not appropriate to close relationships, family or sex relationships. I think it is about boundaries in counselling so that it would be inappropriate for me to take on a student for counselling in its pure sense where I also had another relationship where I also judged the students. That is not to say that I cannot help the students but that I would not take them on for a review of their personal life situation and would recommend that they get their help from someone else.

There are real problems when the client doesn't want counselling. In fact when the individual does not want to be a client. This is a particular problem of people on counselling courses who insist on asking people 'how they feel'. It should not be used as a crowbar for intruding into people's privacy.

The advantages of counselling

Various advantages of counselling were identified by the respondents. One respondent identified its **economic** advantages. He also referred, in passing, to the role of the Church in counselling and the idea of 'counselling as a replacement for a priest'.

It can help you over an immediate crisis or problem. If you are upset you often can't see a way out of a predicament. It's a cheap relative to psychoanalysis or psychotherapy. It is also widely available. A counsellor will give you time in a way that a doctor won't. And for an atheist like myself, a priest is not really an alternative. For a religious person, a priest may be the most appropriate person as the problem may have a spiritual content.

Others found other advantages but often these were **qualified** in various ways suggesting that with the various advantages also came other disadvantages.

My guess that it helps people just to get on with their lives. The fact that I think lots of people can do it. But it does need a willingness and a genuine interest in other human beings which is difficult to 'manufacture'. It can be pretty cheap – a cheap way of helping people. The less formal types of counselling perhaps allow the person who needs the help to maintain some dignity and integrity in the whole process and its not like going to your doctor or going to a psychiatrist because your whole life is falling apart – its sort of more acceptable to society. You can say to people 'I'm going for some counselling' but it is more difficult to say 'I was mentally ill'. There is a greater willingness for people to take counselling on board as acceptable.

[Counselling helps people to have] the opportunity to have a safe situation in which one explores options and choices – particularly where some of those choices may be frightening or where some disclosures of some aspects of ones self may be a presentation of self that one wouldn't want seen elsewhere. If I am looking at a side of myself that I don't want to show to people in every day life but I need to understand, then I may need the confidentiality of a counselling relationship in order to do that.

Sometimes, the view was taken that 'counselling works because people say that it does'.

For the client it would seem to help. I am not sure why. Perhaps I am a bit naive but it seems to help. I've seen it help. And sometimes afterwards I've wondered what I've done that I valued so much and that I missed. I guess that relates to the intuitive nature of counselling if you have counselled for a while.

The disadvantages of counselling

There were also clearly identified **disadvantages** to counselling. Again, these were quite wide-ranging.

It can mislead people into thinking it's a solution, when in fact a real solution may be a material change in the person's circumstances which the counsellor can do nothing to effect. There are a lot of charlatans in counselling. When there is money changing hands the counsellors may have more interest in prolonging the sessions. It is a straightforward market relation sometimes. And like all market relations the profit is a motive and not a human need. The other thing is it is just another way of accommodating oneself to what may be a horrible situation and a better response may be a political one.

One respondent had doubts about the purported practice of teaching student health professionals counselling skills as part of their health care training – arguing that counsellors needed some maturity and some life experience in order to both help the client and to take care of themselves:

One of the things which is true about counselling is that is has become reified – it has become elevated to a supernatural status – particularly in health care. So much so that every curriculum document must have an element of counselling in it. My feeling is that many of the students that I have dealt with are anywhere between 17 and 22 and I do believe that if you're going to be a good counsellor you need to have more life experience as it will help you to put things in perspective. It seems that some courses are expecting to put these young people into counselling and turn them out as mini-counsellors in any arena. I don't think that this is realistic and this is one of the problems as the thing has become more popular. So you have people coming out of courses who will I think have done all these hours of counselling training but these are not underpinned by the years of experience that are needed to be a good counsellor.

Other disadvantages were also noted.

There is the potential opportunity to abuse other people's vulnerability. People do enjoy having power, as experts over people who are very vulnerable and I think this is something to have to guard against.

I would want to distinguish between bad counselling – which one could find quite easily and which could be disempowering and could produce dependency, could mean the person does not own their own decisions. I think there is a continuum in counselling. As counselling gets better the likelihood of those happening are reduced. The good counsellor with a good supervisor would be careful not to let those things happen and would be aware of their propensities to allow those things to happen and would be aware of their own needs to let them happen. In other words the counsellor who gets a buzz out of counselling or enjoys being needed or who wants to take credit for other people's successes is likely to make those disadvantages happen. If one develops as a responsible counsellor one tries to avoid those things. I think we should recognise our own propensity to want to be needed but if we are counselling properly we will look out for that happening.

For the client perhaps, they may feel that it doesn't supply them with any answers. The process can be seen as rather slow or even traumatic.

For the counsellor the disadvantages are that it opens you to an awareness of another person's pain that you may have to avoid due to the situation you are in. And perhaps it can make you weary of other people's distress.

COUNSELLING OR COUNSELLING SKILLS?

A distinction is sometimes made between **counselling** – as an activity carried out by people called counsellors and **counselling skills** – those interpersonal skills that health professionals use to help people. In its *Code of Ethics for Counselling Skills*, the British Association for Counselling states – not always in the clearest terms, the following, as an attempt to clarify what **they** mean by 'counselling skills':

The term 'counselling skills' does not have a single definition which is universally accepted. For the purpose of this code, 'counselling skills' are distinguished from 'listening skills' and from 'counselling'. Although the distinction is not always a clear one, because the term 'counselling skills' contains elements of these other two activities, it has its own place between them. What distinguishes the use of counselling skills from these other two activities are the intentions of the user, which is to enhance the performance of their functional role, as line manager, nurse, tutor, social worker, personnel office, voluntary worker etc., the recipient will, in turn, perceive them in that role (BAC, 1989b).

If there is still a question in the professional's mind, the BAC offers the following questions as a means of clarifying the issue:

1. Are you using counselling to enhance your communication with someone but without taking on the role of their counsellor?
2. Does the recipient perceive you as acting within your professional/caring role (which is **not** that of being their counsellor)?
   (i) If the answer is YES to both these questions, you are using counselling skills in your functional role.
   (ii) If the answer is NO to both, you are counselling and should look to the *Code of Ethics and Practice for Counsellors* for guidance.
   (iii) If the answer is YES to one and NO to the other, you have a conflict of expectations and should resolve it (BAC, 1989b).

The intention of the pointers published by the BAC is, no doubt, to clarify the situation but given the complexity of the range of possible relationships that exist between health care professionals and health care recipients, it seems, to this author, that such a 'step-by-step' means of identifying concrete answers is unlikely to work in the real word. In particular, the second question in the above quotation asks the health professional to 'best guess' the recipient's perceptions of you as a professional. This seems a particularly fraught enterprise as we can rarely know how we are perceived by others short of asking them.

TYPES OF SKILLS

Counselling skills may be divided into three subgroups: (a) introductions, (b) listening and (c) counselling interventions.

Introducing ourselves to others is an important skill. Naming ourselves, describing something of what and who we are is all part of the process of helping the client. The obverse is also true: we need to enable other people to be able to name themselves and to begin to tell their stories. Following an American lead, 'introductions' in the UK are probably handled more skilfully by health professionals than was the case two decades ago. Many health care trusts, for example, have a 'formula' for telephone introductions. Some may feel that the use of a short 'script' in this way is artificial and inauthentic. On the other hand, it is important to give serious consideration to the way in which **you** introduce yourself to other people – both clients and colleagues. This is the case both inside and outside counselling. All health professionals need to pay attention to the issue of how they introduce themselves to others.

Listening has been various defined. Lundsteen suggests that it is 'the process by which spoken language is converted to meaning in the mind' (Lunsteen, 1971). Another, more concrete definition is one offered by Steil who suggests that:

> Listening is the complex, learned human process of sensing, interpreting, evaluating, storing and responding to oral messages (Steil, 1991).

Perhaps, though, we rarely need definitions of listening for all of us have experienced it and know what it is. What is important, though, is that we consider listening fully to the other person.

Listening involves not only giving full attention to the person being listened to but also that we be seen to be listening by the other person. Gerard Egan (1986) argues that in Western countries, the following behaviours are often associated with effective listening and may be practised in order to enhance listening ability.

- **Sit squarely** in relation to the person being listened to. This can be taken both literally and metaphorically. If we are to truly listen to the other person we need to be able to see them and for them to see us, thus it is better that we sit facing them rather than beside them. We also need to 'face' them in the sense of not being put off by them nor daunted by them.
- Maintain an **open** position. Crossed arms and legs can often suggest defensiveness. It is better, then, to sit comfortably and in a relaxed 'uncrossed' position.
- **Lean** slightly towards the person being listened too. Egan argues that this is usually perceived as a warm and interested gesture. On the other hand, it is important that the other person does not feel crowded by the listener.
- Maintain reasonable **eye contact**. The eyes are a potent means of interpersonal communication (Heron, 1970). It is important that our gaze is 'available' for the other person.
- **Relax** while listening. Listening does not have to involve rehearsing the next thing to be said. All that is needed is the listening itself. The relaxed listener helps the person being listened to, to relax.

Egan suggests the acronym SOLER as a means of remembering these basic listening behaviours. The letters in the acronym are used to remember key words in the cycle (in the above descriptions, those keys words have been emboldened).

It should be noted, however, that Egan's behaviours are very probably contextually rooted and – in particular – rooted in the North American culture. There are wide variations, internationally, for example, about the degree to which people do or do not adopt the 'open' position. And regional variations can be considerable. North American men, for example, tend to cross their legs by resting on ankle on the opposite knee. Women in North America and Europe may cross their legs and put their legs 'to one side' when sitting. In Middle and Far Eastern countries, it is often considered bad manners to cross legs at all.

It should also be noted, in passing, that counselling, itself, is very much rooted in a particular culture. Not everyone, in all countries, is going to appreciate the notion of counselling as a helping activity – particularly the client-centred sort. There are many cultures in which seeking advice from a senior member of the culture is far more appropriate than being encouraged to problem-solve, independently.

Eye contact is another regional variable. In a number of cultures, sustained eye contact – particularly between people of different status – is or is not acceptable. Sustained eye contact may be seen as rude or even insulting.

If these things are true of the counsellor and the position that he or she adopts, they also apply to the way in which the client views the counsellor. In other words, the counsellor may have to adapt his or her position and set of behaviours to suit the needs, wants and cultural values of the client.

Listening forms the basis of all good counselling and, arguably, of all interpersonal relationships. If the health profession can learn to enhance her listening ability she will see an improvement in other interpersonal skills, too. Not that listening can ever be a mechanical set of behaviours. It also requires that we are 'present' for the other person: that we are with them as fellow human beings and not purely as professionals doing a job. Rowan offers an analysis of differences between 'ordinary' listening and 'therapeutic' listening (see Table 3.1).

The other sub group of counselling skills is that of counselling interventions: the things that the counsellor says in the counselling relationship. Before specific counselling interventions are discussed, consideration needs to be made of our disposition towards counselling or our 'philosophy' of counselling.

The term 'client-centred', first used by Carl Rogers (1951) refers to the notion that it is the client, himself, who is best able to decide how to find the solutions to their problems in living. 'Client-centred' in this sense may be

Table 3.1 Ordinary listening and therapeutic listening

Ordinary listening	Therapeutic listening
Interest in the content of the statement – what it is intended to convey	Interest in the statement itself as a symptom of things the client did not intend to say
Trying to relate the other person's experience to your own	Not paying attention to your own previous experience
Thinking of interesting replies to carry on the conversation and keep one's end up	Not being concerned with replies or conversations, only with the client's efforts at self-exploration (Rowan, 1983)

contrasted with the idea of 'counsellor-centred' or 'professional-centred', both of which may suggest that someone other than the client is the 'expert'. While this may be true when applied to certain concrete 'factual' problems: housing, surgery, legal problems and so forth, it is difficult to see how it can apply to personal life issues. In such cases, it is the client who identifies the problem and the client who, given time and space, can find their way through the problem to the solution.

Steve Murgatroyd (1986) described the client-centred way of caring as follows:

- a person in need has come to your for help;
- in order to be helped they need to know that you have understood how they think and feel;
- they also need to know that, whatever your own feelings about who or what they are or about what they have or have not done, you accept them as they are – you accept their right to decide their own lives for themselves;
- in the light of this knowledge about your acceptance and understanding of them they will begin to open themselves to the possibility of change and development;
- but if they feel that their association with you is conditional upon them changing, they may feel pressurized and reject your help.

First, the client comes to you for help: not to anyone else. Also, it is not you who comes to the client for help. An obvious point but nevertheless an important one because it highlights the fact that the counsellor/client relationship can never truly be one of equals. The second point is the equally important one that the client needs to be truly understood. The need for empathy – the ability to enter the other person's frame of reference, their view of the world – is essential, here. What we need to consider now are ways of helping the person to express themselves, to open themselves and thus to begin to change. There is an interesting paradox in Murgatroyd's last point: that if the client feels that their association with you is conditional upon them changing, they may reject your help. Thus we enter into the counselling relationship without even being insistent on the other person's changing!

In one sense, this is an impossible position. If we did not hope for change, we presumably would not enter into counselling in the first place! On another level, the point is a very important one. People change at their own rate and in their own time. The process cannot be rushed and we cannot will another person to change (Frankl, 1975). Nor can we expect them to change to become more the sort of person that we would like them to be. We must meet them on their own terms and observe change as they wish and will it to be (or not, as the case may be). This sort of counselling is a very altruistic sort. It demands of us that we make no demands of others.

Client-centred counselling is a process rather than a particular set of skills. It evolves through the relationship that the counsellor has with the client and vice versa. In a sense, it is a period of growth for both parties, for both learn from the other. It also involves the exercise of restraint.

According to counselling orthodoxy, the counsellor must restrain herself from offering advice and from the temptation to 'put the client's life right for him'. Sundeen *et al.* suggest the following problems with advice-giving:

- Advice prevents the client from identifying and pursuing her own chosen course of action.
- Advice blocks the client from exploring emotional issues.
- Advice protects the clinician from feelings of inadequacy.
- Advice leads to premature closure of debate.
- Advice allows the possibility of manipulation of the clinician by the client (Sundeen *et al.*, 1989).

However, it seems likely that idea of **never** offering advice can be overstated. Clearly, all health professionals have information about certain domains that can usefully be shared with clients. It would seem odd, for example, for the doctor or nurse to answer a hospital patient's question about using insulin in the treatment of diabetes: 'what do you feel you should do about insulin?'

It might be argued that advice can be given in concrete, medical situations but not in personal, emotional ones. However, the case is rarely as clear cut as this. There is a danger, perhaps, of the reinvention of the wheel. Most experienced clinicians and practitioners have seen a wide range of human situations in the course of a career. It might seem wasteful and time-consuming always to treat every person's problem as completely new and unique. It seems likely, in this writer's view, that there will be situations in which offering – at least tentative – advice, will be helpful to the client. The keyword, there, is tentative. All advice, perhaps, should be offered as a suggestion, as provisional and as something that might be experimented with.

The outcome of client-centred counselling cannot be predicted nor can concrete goals be set (unless they are devised by the client, at their request). In essence, client-centred counselling involves an act of faith: a belief in the other person's ability to find solutions through the process of therapeutic conversation and through the act of being engaged in a close relationship with another human being.

Assumptions about the client

These, then, are some of the assumptions made about the client-centred approach to counselling. Newell (1994) offers an interesting and useful set of assumptions that may be made about clients in the health care professions. He suggests that the following are useful assumptions to keep in mind when working with clients during interviews and therapy:

- each client is unique;
- each client has skills;

- each client interacts with the environment;
- clients are like us;
- clients are honest;
- each client sincerely desires success;
- each client shares responsibility with the interviewer;
- clients desire interaction and negotiation;
- each client knows what the problem is;
- each client knows when success has occurred (Newell, 1994).

Although Newell's assumptions beg certain questions (**can** we assume that clients are always honest? Can we assume that 'each client knows what the problem is?'), the list offers a useful starting point for thinking about your own assumptions about the people with whom you work.

Client-centred skills

Certain, basic client-centred skills may be identified, although as we have noted, it is the total relationship that is important. Skills exercised in isolation amount to little: the warmth, genuineness and positive regard must also be present. On the other hand, if basic skills are not considered, then the counselling process will probably be shapeless or it will degenerate into the counsellor's becoming prescriptive. The skill of standing back and allowing the client to find his own way is a difficult one to learn. The following interventions or skills may help in the process:

- non-verbal skills;
- questions;
- reflection;
- selective reflection;
- empathy building;
- checking for understanding.

Each of these skill can be learned. In order for that to happen, each must be tried and practised. There is a temptation to say 'I do that anyway!' when reading a description of some of these skills. The point is to notice the doing of them and to practise doing them better! While counselling often shares the characteristics of everyday conversation, if it is to progress beyond that it is important that some, if not all, of the following skills are used effectively and tactfully.

Non-verbal skills

A very large amount of communication between two people takes place on a non-verbal level. It is not just the things that we say to each other that is important, it is also the way we say it. More than this, it is the collection of 'minimal prompts' and hardly discernible behaviours that convey so much. If we counsel someone, we cannot simply rely on being experts at **saying** things, we must also pay attention to all of those other behaviours that fit 'in between' the verbal responses. The following nonverbal responses have been identified as being important:

1. **smiles** used appropriately as indicators of willingness to follow the conversation or pleasure at what the speaker is saying;
2. **direct eye contact**, again to indicate interest in listening to what is being said;
3. indicating enthusiam for the speaker's thoughts and ideas, by using appropriate **paralanguage** when responding (e.g. tone of voice, emphasis on certain words, lack of interruptions of speaker);
4. mirroring the facial **expressions** of the speaker, in order to reflect and express sympathy with the emotional message being conveyed;
5. adopting an attentive **posture**;
6. **nods** of the head to indicate readiness to listen to what the speaker is saying;
7. refraining from distracting mannerisms, such as doodling with a pen, fidgeting or looking at a watch. This is also important in conveying an impression of attention and desire to listen (Hargie, Saunders and Dickson, 1994).

As we have noted, earlier in the chapter, there are huge numbers of tiny, subtle non-verbal forms of communication. We notice, if we are deeply involved in a conversation or a relationship, very slight changes in expression, fleeting movements of the eyes, tiny movements of the mouth and so on. These changes are so varied and numerous that it is probably impossible to produce a typography of them. Also, their meaning differs from person to person and from context to context and from relationship to relationship. Thus a fleeting smile, in one person, may indicate a change of mood, while in another person it indicates a certain hosility. We are faced with a number of imponderables here. First, there is the fact that some subtle forms of non-verbal communication are, presumably, beyond conscious control and, therefore, neither the sender or the receiver can be absolutely clear as to their meaning. Second, there are those non-verbal features that the receiver reads in a certain way and to which he or she attributes certain meanings. Third, there are the meanings intended by the person displaying the subtle non-verbal behaviours. We seem to live out our relationships surrounded by these often confused and confusing non-verbal messages.

QUESTIONS

Two main sorts of questions may be identified in the client-centred approach: closed and open questions. A closed question is one that elicits a 'yes', 'no' or similar one-word answer. Or it is one that the counsellor can anticipate an approximation of the answer, as she asks it. Examples of closed questions are as follows:

- Where do you live?
- Are you married?
- Are you happier now?
- Are you living at home?

Too many closed questions can make the counselling relationship seem like an interrogation! They also inhibit the development of the client's telling of his story and place the locus of responsibility in the relationship firmly with the client. On the other hand, they can be useful in identifying specific information. Three main types of closed questions have been identified:

1. **The selective question**. Here the respondent is presented with two or more alternative responses, from which he is expected to choose.
2. **The yes-no question**. As the name suggests, this is a question that may be adequately answered by a 'yes' or 'no' or by using some equivalent affirmative or negative.
3. **The identification question**. This type of question requires the respondent to identify the answer to a factual question and present this as the response. While the answer to an identification question may involve the recall of information (e.g. 'What is your maiden name?'; 'Where were you born?), it may also be concerned with the identification of present material (e.g. 'What time is it?'; 'Where exactly is the pain occurring now?') or future events (e.g. 'Where are you going on holiday?'; 'When is your baby due?') (Hargie, Saunders and Dickson, 1994).

Open questions

Open questions are those that do not elicit a particular answer: the counsellor cannot easily anticipate what an answer will 'look like'. Examples of open questions include:

- What did you do when that happened?
- How did you feel then?
- How are you thinking right now?
- What do you feel will happen?

Open questions are ones that encourage the client to say more, to expand on their story or to go deeper. Open questions are generally preferable, in counselling, to closed ones. They encourage longer, more expansive answers and are rather more free of value judgements and interpretation than are closed questions. All the same, the counsellor has to monitor the 'slope' of intervention when using open questions. It is easy, for example, to become intrusive by asking too piercing questions, too quickly. As with all counselling interventions, the timing of the use of questions is vital.

Questions can be used in the counselling relationships for a variety of purposes. The main ones include:

- to clarify: 'I'm sorry, did you say you are to move or did you say you're not sure?', 'What did you say then ...?'
- to encourage the client to talk: 'Can you say more about that?', 'What are your feelings about that?'
- To obtain further information: 'How many children have you got?', 'What sort of work were you doing before you retired?'
- To explore: 'What else happened ...?', 'How did you feel then?'

Combining the two

There are pros and cons for using *both* closed and open questions, as we have seen. However, they can often be brought together as 'funnelling'. Funnelling occurs when questions move from the broad to the specific (and, in some cases, when the questions move from the specific to the general). Cohen-Cole and Bird make the following point:

> A considerable body of literature supports the use of open-ended questioning as an efficient and effective vehicle to gain understanding of patients' problems. To be sure, after an initial nondirective phase ... the doctor must ask progressively more focused questions to explore specific diagnostic hypotheses. [This] has been called an 'open-to-closed cone' (Cohen-Cole and Bird, 1991).

Other sorts of questions

There are other ways of classifying questions and some to be avoided! Examples of other sorts of questions including the following:

Leading questions

These are questions that contain an assumption that places the client in an untenable position. The classic example of a leading question is: 'When did you stop beating your wife?'! Clearly, however the question is answered, the client is in the wrong! Other examples of leading questions are:

- Is your depression the thing that's making your work so difficult?
- Are your family upset by your behaviour?
- Do you think that you may be hiding something ... even from yourself?

The later, pseudo-analytical questions are particularly awkward. What could the answer possibly be?

Value-laden questions

Questions such as 'Does your homosexuality make you feel guilty' not only imply a moral judgment but guarantee that the client feels difficult answering them!

'Why' questions

These should always be used sparingly (Schulman, 1982). The 'why' question can easily sound interogative and even moralistic. Also, to ask 'why' about how someone feels is to suggest that they may know why they feel the way they do: this is often not the case. 'Why' questions also lead to a theoretical debate about how the person is feeling. Thus the answer to 'why do you feel depressed?' will always be an offering of that person's theory of why they are depressed. It is often far more useful to discuss the feeling itself.

On the other hand, some have used the 'recursive "why"' as a means of exploring a client's problems in some depth. The process is sometimes known as 'laddering' and can sound like this.

> *Client*: 'I feel depressed at the moment.'
> *Counsellor*: 'Why do you feel depressed?'
> *Client*: 'I don't know. I just don't seem to be able to do anything useful, really.'
> *Counsellor*: 'Why can't you do anything useful?'
> *Client*: 'Because I'm so tired all the time.'
> *Counsellor*: 'Why are you so tired?'
> *Client*: 'Because I'm not sleeping.'
> *Counsellor*: 'Why aren't you sleeping?'
> *Client*: 'I'm worried about what's happening between me and my wife.'
> *Counsellor*: 'What **is** happening?'
> *Client*: 'Well, it started last year ...'

This approach will not suit every counsellor but it can sometimes be a way of getting to the heart of the matter fairly quickly. Used inappropriately, though, it can also be very intrusive and even circular – as in the next example:

> *Client*: 'I'm really feeling depressed at the moment.'
> *Counsellor*: 'Why are you feeling depressed?'
> *Client*: 'Because I'm not sleeping.'
> *Counsellor*: Why aren't you sleeping?'
> *Client*: 'Because I feel so depressed.'

Perhaps this interrogative style of counselling involves the counsellor making an assessment of what a particular client wants and needs from the counsellor. It seems likely that some clients will need space to think things through quietly and with support from the counsellor while others will need a more challenging approach.

Confronting questions

Examples of these may include: 'Can you give me an example of when that happened? and 'Do you still love your wife?'. Confrontation in counselling is quite appropriate once the relationship has fully developed but needs to be used skilfully and appropriately. It is easy for apparent 'confrontation' to degenerate in moralizing. Heron (1986) and Schulman (1982) offer useful approaches to effective confrontation in counselling.

REFLECTION

Reflection (sometimes called 'echoing') is the process of reflecting back the last few words, or a paraphrase of the last few words, that the client has used, in order to encourage them to say more. It is as though the counsellor is echoing the client's thoughts and as though that echo serves as a prompt. It is important that the reflection does not turn into a question and this is best achieved by the counsellor making the repetition in much the same tone of voice as the client used. An example of the use of reflection is as follows:

> *Client*: 'We lived in Edinburgh for a number of months. Then we moved and I supposed that's when things started to go wrong ...'
> *Counsellor*: 'Things started to go wrong ...'

Used skilfully and with good timing, reflection can be an important method of helping the client. On the other hand, if it is overused or used clumsily, it can appear stilted and is very noticeable. Unfortunately, it is an intervention that takes some practice and one that many people anticipate learning on counselling courses. As a result, when people return from counselling courses, their friends and relatives are often waiting for them to use the technique and may comment on the fact! This should not be a deterrent as the method remains a useful and therapeutic one.

SELECTIVE REFLECTION

Selective reflection refers to the method of repeating back to the client a part of something they said that was emphasized in some way or which seemed to be emotionally charged. Thus selective reflection draws from the middle of the client's utterance and not from the end. An example of the use of selective reflection is as follows:

Client: 'I had just started work. I didn't earn very much and I hated the job. Still, it was better than being unemployed, I suppose. It's very difficult these days ...'

Counsellor: 'You hated the job ...'

Client: 'It was the one of the worst periods of my life. I'll never forget working there ...'

The use of selective reflection allowed the client in this example to develop further an almost throwaway remark. Often, these 'asides' are the substance of very important feelings and the counsellor can often help in the release of some of these feelings by using selective reflection to focus on them. Clearly concentration is important, in order to note the points on which to selectively reflect. Also, the counselling relationship is a flowing, evolving conversation that tends to be 'seamless'. Thus, it is little use the counsellor storing up a point that she feels would be useful to selectively reflect! By the time a break comes in the conversation, the item will probably be irrelevant! This points up, again, the need to develop 'free floating attention': the ability to allow the ebb and flow of the conversation to go where the client takes it and for the counsellor to trust her own ability to choose an appropriate intervention when a break occurs.

EMPATHY BUILDING

This refers to the counsellor making statements to the client that indicate that she has understood the feeling that the client is experiencing. A certain intuitive ability is needed here, for often empathy building statements refer more to what is implied than what is overtly said. An example of the use of empathy-building statements is as follows:

Client: 'People at the factory are the same. They're all tied up with their own friends and families ... they don't have a lot of time for me ... though they're friendly enough ...'

Counsellor: 'You sound angry with them ...'

Client: 'I suppose I am! Why don't they take a bit of time to ask me how I'm getting on? It wouldn't take much! ...'

Counsellor: 'It sounds as though you are saying that people haven't had time for you for a long time ...'

Client: 'They haven't. My family didn't bother much ... I mean, they looked as though they did ... but they didn't really ...'

The empathy-building statements, used here, are ones that read between the lines. Now, sometimes such reading between the lines can be completely wrong and the empathy-building statement is rejected by the client. It is important, when this happens, for the counsellor to drop the approach altogether and to pay more attention to listening. Inaccurate empathy-building statements often indicate an overwillingness on the part of the counsellor to become 'involved' with the client's perceptual world – at the expense of accurate empathy! Used skilfully, however, they help the client to disclose further and indicate to the client that they are understood.

CHECKING FOR UNDERSTANDING

Checking for understanding involves either (a) asking the client if you have understood them correctly or (b) occasionally summarizing the conversation in order to clarify what has been said. The first type of checking is useful when the client quickly covers a lot of topics and seems to be 'thinking aloud'. It can be used to further focus the conversation or as a means of ensuring that the counsellor really stays with what the client is saying. The second type of checking should be used sparingly or the counselling conversation can get to seem rather mechanical and studied. The following two examples illustrate the two uses of checking for understanding.

Example (a)

> *Client*: 'I don't know what to do really ... money's OK and I can cope at home ... well, some of the time I can cope at home ... then there's the job. I mean, what do you do?'
>
> *Counsellor*: 'Let me just get things a little more clear ... You say that you don't always cope at home and you don't cope all that well at work ...?'
>
> *Client*: 'Yes ... My parents treat me as though I'm still about 14 and people at work aren't much better!'

Example (b)

> *Counsellor*: 'Let me see if I can just sum up what we've talked about this morning. We talked about your financial problems and the question of seeing the bank manager. You said you may ask him for a loan. Then you went on to say how you felt you could organize your finances better in the future ...?'
>
> *Client*: 'Yes, I think that covers most things ...'

Some counsellors prefer to use the second type of checking at the end of each counselling session and this may help to clarify things before the client leaves. On the other hand, there is much to be said for not 'tidying up' the end of the session in this way. If the loose ends are left, the client continues to think about all the issues that have been discussed, as he walks away from the session. If everything is summarized too neatly, the client may feel that the problems can be 'closed down' for awhile or even worse, that they have been 'solved'! Personal problems are rarely simple enough to be summarized in a few words and the uses of checking at the end of a session should be used sparingly.

These, then, are particular skills that encourage self-direction on the part of the client and can be learned and used by the counsellor. They form the basis of all good counselling and can always be returned to as a primary way of working with the client in the counselling relationship.

LEARNING COUNSELLING SKILLS

Counselling skills can be developed in a variety of ways. Perhaps, for the beginner (if there is such a person!) they are best learned in a small group setting such as the workshop. The essential ingredients of such a workshop, as with other sorts of interpersonal skills workshops are as follows:

1. An adequate theoretical framework. This can be supplied by the workshop facilitator either in the form of a handout, a short lecture or, preferably, through group discussion.
2. Discrimination between different sorts of counselling intervention. The neophyte counsellor needs to be able to choose consciously between different sorts of counselling interventions. Here an analysis such as Heron's (1986) Six Category Intervention Analysis, can be useful. This analysis is described elsewhere in this book.
3. Examples or role models of effective counselling interventions are required. These may be supplied in various ways:
   - the workshop facilitator may model them, in front of the group, with one of the group acting as 'client',
   - the facilitator may do a monodrama and play 'both ends' of a role-play as a demonstration of effective use of counselling interventions,
   - short video films may be used which offer exemplars to the group of effective use of interventions,
   - the facilitator may only describe the interventions and leave the group members to improvise from the descriptions.
4. All the group members need practice in using the interventions. Initially, this practice may take place within the workshop itself. Increasingly, however, the practice should be encouraged away from the workshop setting to encourage reinforcement of the new behaviour in the 'real' situation: the client/health professional relationship.

In the final chapter of this book, a variety of counselling skills exercises are described which will help the facilitator to set up and run a counselling skills workshop. Content for the 'theory' aspect of such a workshop can be gathered from the various titles outlined in the reference section of the book.

It is asserted here that counselling skills are the basic building blocks for skilled interpersonal living. The health professional who can learn to use skilfully a range of counselling skills will find the development of the other interpersonal skills discussed here considerably easier.

ASSERTIVENESS

Assertiveness is often confused with being aggressive. A friend of mine once referred to assertiveness workshops as 'courses for learning how to be rude to other people'! The assertive person is the one who can state clearly and calmly what she wants to say, does not back down in the face of disagreement and is prepared to repeat what she has to say, if necessary. A continuum may be drawn that accounts for a range of types of behaviour ranging from the submissive to the aggressive, with assertive behaviour being the mid point on such a continuum (Figure 3.3). Heron (1986) has argued that when we have to confront another person, we tend to feel anxiety at the prospect. As a result of that anxiety we either tend to 'pussyfoot' (and be submissive) or 'sledgehammer' (and be aggressive). So it is with being assertive. Most people, when they are learning how to assert themselves experience anxiety and as a result tend to be either submissive or aggressive. Other people handle that anxiety by swinging right the way through the continuum. They start submissively, then develop a sort of confidence and rush into an aggressive attack on the other person. Alternatively, some people deal with their anxiety by starting an encounter very aggressively and quickly back off into submission. The level and calm approach of being assertive takes practice, nerve and confidence.

Examples of how assertiveness can be useful include the following situations:

- when used by the client who has never been able to express her wants and needs in a marriage,
- when used by the health professional, when facing bureaucratic processes in trying to get help for her client,
- in everyday situations in shops, offices, restaurants and other places where a stated service being offered is not actually being given.

Arguably, the assertive approach to living is the much clearer one when it comes to dealing with other human beings. The submissive person often loses friends because they come to be seen as duplicitous, sycophantic or as a 'doormat'. On the other hand, the aggressive person is rarely popular perhaps, simply, because most of us don't particularly like aggression. The assertive person comes to be seen as an 'adult' person who is able treat other people reasonably and without recourse to either childish or loutish behaviour. Much has been written about the topic of assertiveness and the reader is referred to the recommended reading list at the end of this volume.

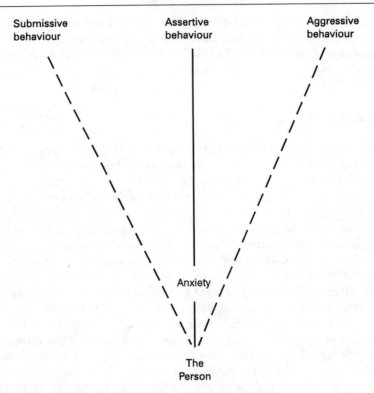

Figure 3.3 A continuum of assertive and non-assertive behaviours

Alberti and Emmons (1982) identify four major elements in assertive behaviour:

1. intent: the assertive person does not intend to be hurtful to others by stating his own needs and wants;
2. behaviour: behaviour classified as assertive would be evaluated by an 'objective observer' as honest, direct, expressive and non-destructive of others;
3. effects: behaviour classified as assertive has the affect on the other of a direct and non-destructive message by which that person would not be hurt;
4. socio-cultural context: behaviour classified as assertive is appropriate to the environment and culture in which it is demonstrated and may not necessarily be considered 'assertive' in a different socio-cultural environment.

Thus Alberti and Emmons invoke some ethical dimensions to the issue of assertiveness. They are suggesting that, used correctly, assertive behaviour is not intended to hurt the other person, should not be perceived as being hurtful and that assertive behaviour is dependent upon culture and context. They further suggest that assertive behaviour can be broken down into at least the following components.

Eye contact

The assertive person is able to maintain eye contact with another person to an appropriate degree.

Body posture

The degree of assertiveness that we use is illustrated through our posture, the way in which we stand in relation to another person and the degree to which we face the other person squarely and equally.

Distance

There seems to be a relationship between the distance we put between ourselves and another person and the degree of comfort and equality we feel with that person. If we feel overpowered by the other person's presence, we will tend to stand further away from them than we would do if we felt equal to them. Proximity in relation to others is culturally dependent but, in a common-sense way, we can soon establish the degree to which we, as individuals, tend to stand away from others or feel comfortable near to them.

Gestures

Alberti and Emmons suggest that appropriate use of hand and arm gestures can add emphasis, openness and warmth to a message and can thus emphasize the assertive approach. Lack of appropriate hand and arm gestures can suggest lack of self-confidence and lack of spontaneity.

Facial expression / tone of voice

It is important that the assertive person is congruent in their use of facial expression (Bandler and Grinder, 1975). Congruence is said to occur when what a person says is accompanied by an appropriate tone of voice and by appropriate facial expressions. The person who is incongruent may be perceived as unassertive. An example of this is the person who says he is angry but smiles as he says it: the result is a mixed and confusing communication.

Fluency

A person is likely to be perceived as assertive if he is fluent and smooth in his use of his voice. This may mean that those who frequently punctuate their conversation with 'ums' and 'ers' are perceived as less than assertive.

Timing

The assertive person is likely to be able to pay attention to his 'end' of a conversation. He will not excessively interrupt the other person, nor will he be prone to leaving long silences between utterances.

Listening

As was noted about the effective counsellor, the assertive person is likely to be a good listener. The person who listens effectively not only has more confidence in his ability to maintain a conversation but also illustrates his interest in the other person. Being assertive should not be confused with being self-centred.

Content

Finally, it is important that what is said is appropriate to the social and cultural situation in which a conversation is taking place. Any English person who has been to America will know about the unnerving silence that is likely to descend on a conversation if he uses words such as 'fag' or 'lavatory' in certain settings! So will the person who uses slang or swear words in inappropriate situations. It is important, in being perceived as assertive, that a person learns to use appropriate words and phrases.

A paradox emerges out of all these dimensions of assertive behaviour. The assertive person also has to be genuine in his presentation of self. Now if that person is too busy noticing his behaviour and verbal performance, he is likely to feel distinctly self-conscious and contrived. It would seem that assertiveness training, like other forms of interpersonal skills training, tends to go through three stages and an understanding of those stages can help to resolve that paradox.

- Stage one: The person is unaware of his behaviour and unaware of the possible changes that he may bring about in order to become more assertive.
- Stage two: The person begins to appreciate the various aspects of assertive behaviour, practises them and temporarily becomes clumsy and self-conscious in their use.
- Stage three: The person incorporates the new behaviours into his personal repertoire of behaviours and 'forgets' them but is perceived as more assertive. The new behaviours have become a 'natural' part of the person.

It is asserted that if behaviour change in interpersonal skills training is to become relatively permanent, the person must learn to live through the rather painful second stage of the above model. Once through it, the new skills become more effective as they are incorporated into that person's everyday presentation of self. Zuker (1983) goes as far as to offer a general Assertive Bill of Rights, which includes the rights to:

- be treated with respect;
- have and express personal feelings and opinions;
- be listened to and taken seriously;
- set one's own priorities;
- say no without feeling guilty;
- ask for what one wants;
- get what one pays for;

- make mistakes;
- assert oneself even though it may inconvenience others;
- choose not to assert oneself.

This does, of course, raise various questions. Do we really have these as 'rights'? Can we expect others to respect these conditions and what if they do not? Are they asserting their own rights to act as they please? The Bill of Rights could be seen as encouraging people to be rather too demanding and too self-centred.

Also, as is the case with client-centred counselling, assertiveness is very much rooted in particular cultures – mostly those of the USA and Northern Europe. In other countries and other cultures, the idea that people should be assertive is not one readily ascribed to. We should be careful about assuming that assertiveness is necessarily an appropriate form of behaviour and be wary about 'inflicting' it on people from other cultures. This is particularly important in the current educational climate in health care in which university departments are often contracted to teach in other parts of the world. It is easy to assume, unthinkingly, that what suits a British or American health care group will suit an audience in the Middle or Far East. This is often far from being the case. It is important for the interpersonal skills trainer, visiting other countries, to learn as much as possible about the culture before making assumptions. A number of years ago, I taught client-centred counselling skills to a group of health care professionals in a Muslim country. The week seemed to have gone well but, on the last day, a senior participant in the group asked me:

> 'Why do you bother with this "client-centred" approach? Nothing that you or I can do will make any difference. Allah will sort everything out one way or the other. We accept that: you still think that **individuals** will make a difference.'

LEARNING TO BE ASSERTIVE

In developing assertiveness in others, the trainer is clearly going to have to be able to role model assertive behaviour herself. The starting point in this field, then, is personal development if it is required. This can be gained through attendance, initially, at an assertiveness training course and later through undertaking a 'training the trainers' course. There are an increasing number of colleges and extra-mural departments of universities which offer such courses and they are also often included in the list of topics offered as evening courses.

Once the trainer has developed some competence in being assertive, the following stages need to be followed in the organization of a successful training course for others:

- Stage One: A theory input which explains the nature of assertive behaviour, including its differentiation from submissive and aggressive behaviour.
- Stage Two: A discussion of the participants' own assessment of their assertive skills or lack of them. This assessment phase may be enhanced by volunteers role-playing typical situations in which they find it difficult to be assertive.
- Stage Three: Examples of assertive behaviour from which the participants may role-model. These may be offered in the form of short video film presentations, demonstrations by the facilitator with another facilitator, demonstrations by the facilitator with a participant in the workshop or through demonstrations offered by skilled people invited into the workshop to demonstrate assertive behaviour. The last option is perhaps the least attractive as too good a performance can often lead to group participants feeling deskilled. It is easy for the less confident person to feel 'I could never do that'. For this reason, too, it is important that the facilitator running the workshop does not present herself as being too assertive but allows some 'faults' to appear. A certain amount of lack of skill in the facilitator can be, paradoxically, reassuring to course participants.
- Stage Four: Selection, by participants, of situations that they would like to practise in order to become more confident in being assertive. Commonly requested situations, here, may include:
  - responding assertively to a marriage partner;
  - dealing with colleagues at work more assertively;
  - returning faulty goods to shops or returning unsatisfactory food in a restaurant;
  - not responding aggressively in a discussion;
  - being able to speak in front of a group of people or deliver a short speech.

These situations can then be rehearsed using the slow role-play method, described above. At each stage of the role-play, the participants are encouraged to reflect on their performances and adopt assertive behaviour if they have slipped into being either aggressive or submissive. Sometimes, this means replaying the role-play several times.

- Stage Five: Carrying the newly learned skills back into the 'real world'. Sometimes, the very act of having practised being assertive is enough to encourage the person to practise being assertive away from the workshop. More frequently, however, there needs to be a follow-up day or a series of follow-up days in which progress, or lack of it, is discussed and further reinforcement of effective behaviour is offered.

In Chapter 9, a series of activities for encouraging the development of assertive behaviour is offered. These activities may be used throughout the type of workshop described here.

Acquiring interpersonal skills in professional life | 4

In previous chapters we have considered the nature of experiential learning, experiential learning methods and some of the interpersonal skills that may be learned by the experiential approach. What is also necessary is that we as students and as professional health care workers learn to pay attention to how our skills are changing and developing. In this chapter a variety of methods of acquiring and enhancing skills are discussed and particular attention is paid to two concrete and practical methods of recording and enhancing interpersonal competence: the journal and the mentor system.

ACQUIRING INTERPERSONAL SKILLS

The most obvious methods of monitoring progress in interpersonal skills development have been discussed already: (a) practising the skills involved and (b) noticing our changing and developing reactions. The practice element often comes with the job. We are involved in interpersonal relationships every day of our professional lives so there is plenty of time for trying out new behaviour. It has to be noted, however, that the decision to try out new interpersonal behaviour must be a conscious one. It is very easy to attend a workshop on counselling skills and to believe that a lot was gained from it. The truth is of course that the workshop will only have been successful if the learning gained in it is transferred to the 'real' situation. There is always a danger of an interpersonal skills workshop being an 'island' in the middle of a busy working life – something that was interesting at the time, but of little practical value. The practical value will only be evident if the transfer of learning occurs. This point is an important one for those who facilitate experiential learning workshops. They must attempt to ensure that learning is carried over into real life and does not remain within the confines of the comfortable atmosphere of the workshop. To this end, some facilitators use 'homework' as a means of reinforcing learning.

Others ask workshop participants to set personal contracts with themselves to try out new learning. Others, still, have follow-up days on which all the participants meet again and discuss their progress or lack of it.

The second point is a reminder about the concept of 'noticing'. We need not only to practise new behaviour but also to reflect on what effect it has both on ourselves and on the recipients of that behaviour. As we noted in the previous chapters, it is important to practise the skill of noticing – of having our attention rooted firmly in the present, of paying attention to ourselves and to our surroundings. As with many of these personal skills, the only way to develop the skill of noticing is to do it! Try it now and continue to notice throughout the day. If you forget and your attention wanders, slowly allow it to return and keep trying!

In summary, there are three basic requirements for 'formally' developing interpersonal competence:

- attendance at a training course or workshop;
- practice of new interpersonal skills in the real situation;
- continuing ability to notice what happens to us and other people when we use interpersonal skills.

We also learn new skills incidentally through a trial and error process and we also need to monitor our progress of interpersonal growth. The two methods, alluded to above, for undertaking that monitoring – keeping a journal and using the mentor system – are now described. These methods can help us to maintain and evaluate both formal and informal learning.

KEEPING A JOURNAL

There is a growing literature on the use of self and peer assessment on the interpersonal skills field (Kilty, 1978; 1982; Burnard, 1987). With the increase in interest in experiential learning is coming the realisation that those taking part in interpersonal workshops and in various forms of experiential learning need to be able to develop their own criteria for checking and evaluating their own learning (Knowles, 1975; 1978; 1980). In this section, the use of one such student-centred approach is discussed: the journal as a method of self-assessment and evaluation.

It is acknowledged that the two concepts of assessment and evaluation are linked. To assess is to identify a particular state at particular time, usually with a view to taking action to change or modify that state. To evaluate is to place a value on a course of action, to identify the success or otherwise of something that has happened. Thus assessment is often seen as something that needs to occur at the outset of an educational encounter and evaluation something that occurs at the end. In fact, evaluation necessarily leads on to reassessment and thus to another educational encounter. In this way the journal described here can be used both as an assessment tool and as an evaluation instrument.

A modified version of the journal has been used at the School of Nursing Studies, University of Wales College of Medicine, as part of a continuous assessment procedure during the Bachelor of Nursing course, during students' mental health nursing secondment. It has met with varying amounts of success. After an initial period of the students' feeling that they would not be able to complete the journal, a number found it particularly useful and planned to continue to use it throughout other parts of their course. Others continued to find it difficult to use and one never completed it.

The instructions for completion of the journal are simple. Participants are required to make weekly entries in a suitable book under the following headings:

- problems encountered and resolution of those problems;
- application of new skills and difficulties with them;
- new skills required to be learned;
- personal growth issues/self awareness development;
- other comments.

These headings can be varied according to the needs and wants of a particular group using the journal approach. No guidelines need to be given regarding the amount that is written under each heading. To prescribe a particular number of words would be over-structuring, although it may be possible to negotiate maxima and minima with the group.

Participants are encouraged to make regular entries and this regularity tends to make the process of keeping the diary easier. Participants who try to 'catch up' and complete the whole thing in one last go tend to have difficulty in remembering what has happened and generally the process is less valuable.

There are several methods of using the diary as an assessment/evaluation tool. The first is to use it as a continuous focus of discussion between the facilitator and the group, in an on-going group. In this way, the participants' experience is constantly being monitored and they are able to discuss their progress or lack of it as they continue with day-to-day fieldwork.

The second method is to use it as a means of summative evaluation at the end of a period of fieldwork (Scriven, 1967). In this case, the following procedure may be used:

- Both facilitator and student sit down and individually 'brainstorm' criteria for assessing the journal. Examples of items brainstormed may be:
  - quality of writing,
  - clarity of expression,
  - ability to problem-solve,
  - level of self-disclosure, etc.
- After this brainstorming session, both facilitator and participant identify three criteria that they wish to use as criteria for assessing the journal.

- Each then uses those criteria to write notes on their assessment of the journal and then compare those notes.

Out of this activity comes a shared view of the journal that incorporates elements of both self and facilitator evaluation. The discussion that follows can be useful to both participants and facilitator as a means of offering further feedback on performance. This method can also be used to focus on another important communication skill, the written word. This is a particularly fruitful area if the participant is, in this case, a student or trainee in the health care field. At this stage, too, a mark for the diary can be negotiated if the journal is to form part of a continuous assessment procedure.

A third method of using the journal is as part of a weekly discussion. This can serve as a means of focusing on shared problems and also as a method of disseminating new information and learning. The journal can also form the basis of a seminar group, with each member in turning taking the lead to run the group.

Probably the most democratic method of deciding upon how to use the journal is to negotiate that use with the group. This should be done prior to the journal being undertaken so that all participants are clear as to who will and who will not have access to it. Journal writing calls for a considerable degree of self-disclosure and it is important, in adult learning groups, that the participants' dignity is maintained (Jarvis, 1983).

The journal as part of a total assessment and evaluation system in an interpersonal skills training course or as part of a larger training course can be a valuable and very personal means of participants' maintaining a constant check on their own learning and development. The approach can be modified in a variety of ways to reflect different emphases. For instance, the bias can be towards practical skills development, or towards self-awareness. Alternatively, participants can be encouraged to develop their own headings for the journal in order to reflect their own needs and wants.

It is interesting to consider the various levels of assessment and evaluation that take place when this method is used. First, the participants have to reflect on their experience before they write. Second, they have to covert their thoughts into words and write an entry in the journal. Third, another level of assessment occurs when the journal is discussed between other group members or in a tutorial. In this way, participants are completing part of the experiential learning cycle discussed in Chapter 1. They are also fulfilling the conditions of self-disclosure and feedback from others that Luft (1969) considers necessary for the development of self-awareness. Thus the method offers a valuable educational tool on a number of levels.

Redwine (1989) develops the idea of a diary further when she advocates encouraging students to write an **autobiography**. She suggests that this written document can then be shared between members of a learning group and that the sharing does at least three things:

- It acts as a catharsis and helps the students deal with many areas in their lives that they have not dealt with. Because of the very nature of the students, there are many commonalities. They dropped out of school and got married and/or started working. They had problems with parents as teenagers; they often have low self-esteem ...
- It binds the group together and forms a support group for the next year when they are studying independently. A call or a letter to or from a fellow seminar participant is always encouraging.
- It serves as a basis for credit for particular aspects of their experiential learning. As the participants relive their lives, they recall learning experiences they might not otherwise have thought of (Redwine, 1989).

For those who are teaching extended interpersonal skills courses, this would seem to be an area of useful exploration.

ACQUIRING INTERPERSONAL SKILLS IN THE HEALTH PROFESSIONS: NUMBER 9

Attending workshops

Try to attend workshops on interpersonal skills training on a regular basis even if you are a trainer yourself. You will see other people facilitating groups and learn new ideas.

SUPERVISION AND THE MENTOR SYSTEM

In learning and developing interpersonal skills we all need help at times. Sometimes it is useful if the help regularly comes from the same person and we can develop a lasting relationship with that helper. It is here that we find the basis of the notion of mentoring. The idea of having a mentor during health care training received considerable attention in the American press (Atwood, 1979; May *et al.*, 1982) and two writers go as far as to say that 'everyone who makes it has a mentor' (Collins and Scott, 1979). Burton (1977) notes that many of the famous American playwrights and poets revealed that they had mentors at some stage in their careers. In this country, the notion has been less written about but is gaining momentum in the health care professions as a format for developing interpersonal skills in health professionals. In Torbay Health Authority (Johns and Morris, 1988) for example, the mentor relationship has been used with considerable success in working out a new style of psychiatric nurse education.

What, then, is a mentor, why do we need them and how do we train them? A mentor is usually someone older than the student and who has considerable experience of the job for which the student is being prepared. The idea of having a mentor also usually contains the idea of continuity and of the student's staying with the mentor for some time. This is in contrast to more traditional approaches to health professionals' education, where continuity with teaching staff is necessarily interrupted by field experience and where students work with a qualified person for only a short period of time. With the mentor system, trainees negotiate who their mentor will be and then stay 'allocated' to that person for the length of their training. Necessarily, then, a closer relationship is likely to develop between the mentor and student than has traditionally been the case.

Darling (1984) found in her research that there were three 'absolute requirements for a significant mentoring relationship'. These were: attraction, action and affect. In the first instance, attraction, it is deemed vital that both people respect and like each other. Arguably, as the relationship develops, a transference relationship will evolve (Burton, 1977). The term transference is usually reserved as a descriptor for the nature of the relationship that develops between a psychotherapist and her client. It signifies that the client comes to see the therapist as having personal characteristics (usually positive ones) that are reminiscent of one of the client's parents. All this normally takes place at a pre or unconscious level so the client does not readily see that this is happening. The net result is usually that the client 'idealizes' the therapist and becomes very dependent on her. One of the aims of therapy is often to help the client to try to resolve this transference relationship and thus live a less dependent and more interdependent life (Burnard, 1989). It seems likely that the relationship between student and mentor is also likely to invoke transference, particularly as the mentor is already cast in the role of 'expert' by the very nature of being a mentor at all. All this suggests that mentors should be choosen very carefully. Who should do this 'choosing' remains a question for debate!

It is possible, too, that the 'attraction' could include emotional and sexual attraction. The ethical position, here, is clear – at least in theory. The relationship between mentor and student should remain a 'Platonic' one, given the tacit contract that exists between teachers, clinical staff and students. Life is rarely as simple as that, however, and the issue of how to cope with more involved relationships clearly needs addressing.

In terms of the 'action' role of the mentor, the student is likely to want to use the mentor as a role model. Again, by definition, the mentor is seen as an expert: someone who has achieved the various skills that are deemed necessary for effective practice and who is able to use and pass on those skills. In a sense, this aspect of mentoring may be equivalent to the 'sitting with Nellie' approach to training office staff in some organizations. 'Sitting with Nellie' refers to the idea of learning skills by sitting with and watching the person who has them. Clearly, though, it is to be hoped that this will not be the only way that skills are passed on. Traditionally, there has been an element of this approach in the past training approaches for students. Just being with a qualified person was sometimes seen as enough to encourage and enable students to develop skills.

Whether or not this was ever the case is another debatable point! A certain skill in coaching seems to be a requirement of the skilled mentor. The ability to break down skills into component parts and teach them and then the ability to demonstrate their use with the appropriate, accompanying effect, seems to be another skill to aim for. Mentoring, it would seem, is not for the faint-hearted!

From the 'affective' point of view, the mentor needs to act in a supportive role. She should be able to encourage the student, enhance her self-confidence and teach her to be constructively critical of what she sees and does. Again, this aspect of the role is likely to re-open the debate about the likelihood of a transference relationship occurring. If it does and transference does occur, it is important that the mentor will be able to cope with it. She will also need to know how to close the relationship and be skilled in 'saying goodbye'. This is unlikely to be easy because of the possible 'counter-transference' that may occur: the mentor's complicated network of feelings for the student! At best, however, the relationship may come to mirror the best aspects of the truly therapeutic relationship that the student will develop with her patients. Hopefully, then, the mentor will be able to initiate and sustain the sort of exemplary relationship that will stand as a role model for future relationships. Again, a lot is being asked of the person who acts as mentor.

If such a relationship does develop and is sustained, it is likely to be very valuable for the student and, no doubt, for the mentor. If the heart of nursing is concerned with relationships, then a close relationship between one who 'knows' and one who is learning may be useful to both and, subsequently, to the patients.

On the other hand, there are numerous problems. Because of the nature of the partnership, the student starts in a 'one-down' relationship with the mentor.The mentor is necessarily in a dominant position in the relationship. It is not and cannot be a relationship of equals. Now much of the recent writing on adult education has suggested that adult education should concern itself with negotiation, with shared learning and with meeting students' own perceived needs (Brookfield, 1987). The adult, so this argument goes, needs to use what they learn, as they learn it; they need to be treated as equals in a partnership that leads along a road of enquiry; they need to have their self-concept protected, as they go. Now whether such demands for equality and negotiation can exist within the constraints of the mentor/student relationship is not clear. It seems more likely that the mentor will be identified as a benign (or perhaps, not so benign!) father or mother substitute. Some may find such a portrayal overdramatic, but, as we have noted, the perfectly respectable notion of transference depends upon the 'unconscious designation' of the other person as a surrogate parent.

There is also the problem of the mentor's own development. There is nothing worse than the 'guru' who feels that she has gained enlightenment and all she needs to do is to sit back and pass on pearls of wisdom to others! I write 'she': unfortunately, such guru figures are nearly always male! All of us need to continue our development and education. None of us has 'arrived'; none of us is skilled to the point where we cannot learn other skills. The mentor must be a convert, if to anything, to lifelong education (Gross, 1977, Mocker and Spear, 1982).

Lifelong education is a concept that fits in well with the notion of experiential learning. With lifelong learning the assumption is that education does not and should not end with 'formal' education. Unfortunately, the preparation of many health care professionals is such that a 'front-end' model of education and training is offered. That is to say that there is a lengthy preparation period (often of between two and six years) followed by very little further education, apart from the occasional study day. The responsibility for further and continuing education thus becomes the responsibility of the individual practitioner. This is particularly pertinent to the mentor who will be responsible for helping the newcomer to the profession. Lifelong learning commends an approach entailing personal responsiblility for learning. Ronald Gross, in his introductory text *The Lifelong Learner* sums up this approach as follows:

> This idea of self-development is the link between your life and learning. A free learner seizes the exhilarating responsibility for the growth of his or her own mind. This starts when you realise that you must decide what you will make of yourself (Gross, 1977).

Lifelong learning is concerned with growth and development. There are echoes, here, of Whitehead's (1933) remark, quoted in the first chapter of this book: 'knowledge keeps no better than fish!'. The lifelong learner is one who does not hoard 'dead knowledge' but appreciates the changing nature of it. What serves us well as knowledge and skill, today, will to quite an extent be out of date tomorrow. No health professional can afford to allow her knowledge and skills base to become out of date. Interestingly, the task of being a mentor can help in the process of keeping up to date, for the mentor also learns from the person for whom she is mentor.

This raises an interesting paradox. While the mentor takes reponsibility for overseeing the learner, she must also be constantly consulting that learner about how he or she will determine the next part of his or her learning. The mentor, in other words, should always be trying to do herself out of a job.

All of these things, and no doubt plenty more, need consideration before the partnership of mentoring begins. Alternatively, they could be faced as they occur, which may be the more painful way.

How can mentors be trained? Should they be trained? There is a tendency, in some quarters, to be disparaging about training in the interpersonal domain. Some prefer to think of health professionals as having 'natural' ability in their field. It would seem reasonable, however, to try to identify some of the aspects of the role that would lend themselves to training.

First, the mentor will need skills in identifying learning objectives, with the student. This involves skilful negotiation of the student's objectives. Such negotiation takes two factors into account: (1) what the student identifies as a need and (2) what the mentor identifies as a need. Together, the two people must work out a reasonable and workable programme.

Second, the mentor will need to be interpersonally competent. By this I mean that they will be able to initiate and maintain a student-centred relationship that takes full account of the possibility of transference occurring. They will be skilled as a counsellor and be prepared to set aside a regular time to talk to the student. This aspect of the role may be described as the 'befriending' aspect.

Thirdly, they will need coaching skills. They will require the ability, described above, to encourage learning. This is, of course, different to the skills required of a teacher, for mentors will not be teachers in the traditional sense of that term. Students will, however, by various means, learn a great deal from them!

Finally, in this tentative list of requirements, the mentor will need skills in enabling the student to self-evaluate – both the student's skills and the nature of the mentor/student relationship. Thus the mentor will be encouraging the development of self-awareness in the student. Such awareness is likely to help the student in their subsequent relationships with patients or clients. Generally, the relationship needs to be an unselfish one on the part of the mentor.

These are two important methods of evaluating and monitoring experience. Both are non-traditional methods and both offer the health professional who is learning to develop interpersonal competence the tools to develop their awareness and to identify new learning goals.

5 | Educational principles and curriculum design in experiential learning

All educational activities are underpinned by certain philosophical beliefs about the nature of education. This chapter explores two approaches to education and offers a practical example of one approach in action. In discussing the broad principles behind the experiential learning approach and considering the work of adult educators, the reader will be able to make considerations about how to plan workshop and course programmes with rather than for the participants. The chapter paves the way towards a discussion of the specific skills of the facilitation of experiential workshops for interpersonal skills training.

While training and educational methods in the health care professions vary, many of them support a traditional notion of learning. It is worth considering, for example, how much time is devoted, in your own branch of the health field, to the following aspects of interpersonal skills:

- counselling;
- group facilitation;
- self-awareness;
- coping with client's and patient's emotional release (tears, anger, fear, embarrassment).

If they are dealt with at all, how are they covered? As a lecture, a discussion or experientially?

THE CURRICULUM

The term 'curriculum' has been variously defined by educationalists. Skilbeck, for example, identified four ways of thinking about the curriculum:

1. curriculum as a structure of forms and fields of knowledge;
2. curriculum as a character map of the culture;

ACQUIRING INTERPERSONAL SKILLS IN THE HEALTH PROFESSIONS: NUMBER 10

Sculpting

Ask for group members to volunteer an example of an encounter with a client that did not go well. Then allow the person who volunteers the encounter to describe it to the group. Then invite a few group members to recreate the scene and to 'freeze' their postures and non-verbal behaviours.

When all group members have had the chance to observe the 'sculpt', facilitate a discussion about it.

---

3. curriculum as a pattern of learning activities;
4. curriculum as a learning technology (Skilbeck, 1984).

All of these approaches apply to the one taken in this book. As we have noted in the first chapter, various forms of knowledge – propositional, practical and experiential – are all part of the experiential approach to teaching interpersonal skills. The 'culture' aspect of Skilbeck's approach mirrors the notion, in this book, that teaching interpersonal skills can involve considering prevailing and personal values. Experiential learning activities constitute the 'pattern' element of Skilbeck's list and the experiential approach may be considered a form of 'learning technology'.

Taking a broader approach to defining curriculum, Quinn offers a practical checklist of features that he argues constitute the concept of curriculum and these are of value to any health care trainer who is considering how to plan interpersonal skills training:

- Who is to be taught? Who will learn? This is the **consumer** of the curriculum, i.e. the student, course member, colleague, etc. who will experience the curriculum.
- What is to be taught and/or learned? This is about both the **intentions** and the **content** of the curriculum. Intentions may or may not be stated overtly, according to the educational ideology underpinning the curriculum. Where outcomes, goals, or objectives are overtly expressed, these statements also indicate to some extent the nature of the curriculum content. If the intentions are covert, then content is usually indicated by a list of topics in a syllabus.
- Why is it to be taught and/or learned? This is the **ideology** of the curriculum, i.e. the teaching, learning and assessment approaches or opportunities available to the consumer.
- Where is it to be taught/learned? This is the **context** of the curriculum, i.e. the faculty, department, school, college, campus, rooms, etc. It also refers to the place of a given curriculum within a range of awards of the educational provider institution.

- When is it to be taught and/or learned? This is the **programming/ timetabling** of the curriculum, i.e. the length, pattern of attendance etc. (Quinn, 1995).

TWO APPROACHES TO EDUCATION AND LEARNING

The approach to learning suggested in this book suggests a certain view of education. This view is best articulated by a series of comparisons between two types of curriculum models. The two types are illustrated in Table 5.1. The table offers two 'ideal types' of curriculum, the classical and the romantic. This distinction has been made by a variety of writers, including the novelist, Robert Pirsig (1974) and the educationalist, Dennis Lawton (1973), who uses them to make comparisons between types of curricula in a similar manner to that described here.

It is suggested that the two curriculum models offer two different views of the nature of education and a closer examination of the two may help to illustrate this. The classical model is teacher or tutor-centred: the teacher is the more important figure than the learner in that they plan and execute the programme. The teacher is the 'one who knows' and the student as the 'one who comes to learn'. The romantic model, on the other hand is student-centred and its main aim is learning. In this model the teacher acts as a resource or as a 'facilitator of learning' (Rogers, 1983). A facilitator is not a teacher but one who helps others to learn for themselves.

Table 5.1 Two models of education and of the curriculum

	Classical curriculum	Romantic curriculum
Focus of the educational encounter	Teacher-centred	Student-centred
Aim of the educational process	Teaching	Learning
Aims and objectives	Set by teacher	Negotiated
Content of the curriculum	Decided by teacher	Evolve out of relationship between teacher and learner
Learning methods	Didactic, lecture centred	Activity, experience based
Evaluation	Exams set by teacher or examining board	Self and peer evaluation
Nature of knowledge	Absolutist: facts are objective	Relativist: knowledge involves personal perceptions

The romantic model is more in keeping with the experiential learning approach discussed in this book. For that reason it is worth exploring, further, the differences between the two curriculum approaches. The health professional who uses a particular model for teaching interpersonal skills needs to have considered her underlying values and beliefs about education if she is to be consistent in her practice. Later on, we will explore the practical implications of some of these issues.

In the classical model, aims and objectives are predetermined by the teacher. Lessons are pre-planned independently of the students. In the romantic model, aims and objectives are negotiated with the learners: students' needs and wants are identified and then learning sessions are developed around those needs and wants.

In the classical model, teaching methods are also pre-determined by the teacher. In the romantic model they are chosen through collaboration with the learners and participation in the learning process is voluntary. There is also, usually, an accent on activity: the learner is encouraged to take an active part in her own learning process.

Evaluation of learning, in the classical model, is by tests and examinations set by the teacher or by an outside examining board. In the romantic model both facilitator and learners engage in self and peer-evaluation (Kilty, 1982; Burnard, 1987). These approaches to evaluation enable the learner to assess her own performance and to receive feedback from both the facilitator and the other people in her learning group. In this way, she receives a 'triangulated' form of evaluation: she has three sets of perceptions of her learning, instead of one.

It may be noted that the classical model involves 'teaching from above' while the romantic model is more concerned with the 'education of equals' (Jarvis, 1983). In the romantic model, students and facilitator are 'fellow travellers', for, as we saw in the diagram, the view of knowledge offered in this model is relative. There are no absolute truths or facts but views of the world are negotiated through discussion, argument and debate. Because each person's view of the world is different, so individual people's 'knowledge' will be different. In the classical model, knowledge is not relative: there are objective facts out there in the world that are subject to apprehension by those who seek them – a view of knowledge that can be traced back at least to Plato. It is the teacher's task, within this model, to pass on those objective facts. In the classical model, knowledge is 'impartial' and is unchanged by the one who knows it (Peters, 1969). In the romantic model, knowledge is dynamic and ever-changing and very much a part of the one who does the knowing.

A similar distinction between two approaches to education is made by Paulo Freire (1972) who described the 'banking' concept of education versus the 'problem-posing' concept. The banking concept (which Freire argues is the traditional and predominant one) involves the teacher's helping to fill her students with knowledge, which is later 'cashed out', relatively unchanged, in examinations. In this model, 'more knowledge' is usually synonymous with 'better educated'. Alternatively, Freire's problem-posing approach to education is a means of education through dialogue. Facilitator and students meet and exchange ideas and experiences through critical argument and debate. Neither facilitator nor student has the 'right' answer: there is room for 'multiple realities' – different views of the world built on different experiences of that world.

Blaney (1974) summarizes the more traditional teaching and learning relationship through reference to a variety of typical criteria, including the following.

- Authority is assumed by the educational institution and is largely external to the learners.
- Objectives are determined prior to the educational encounter, and these provide the basis for program planning and evaluation. These objectives are consonant with the aims of the providing agency, although they may be revised by the teacher.
- Methods of instruction are chosen for their demonstrated effectiveness in achieving the previously determined objectives.
- The teacher's roles are those of instructional planner, manager of instruction, diagnostician, motivator and evaluator.
- The learner assumes a dependent role regarding learning objectives and evaluative criteria; the learner's task is to achieve the prescribed objectives.
- Evaluation is criterion referenced, and criteria are based on the achievement of the prescribed objectives. The purpose of evaluation is to assess the effectiveness of instruction in assisting learners to achieve the prescribed objectives, to improve the program, and to diagnose learning difficulties.

It is interesting to ponder on the degree to which education and training in the health care professions is organized within such criteria!

ADULT LEARNING

The American adult learning theorist, Malcolm Knowles, cites Lindeman (1926) as the source of the following 'foundation stones of modern adult learning theory' (Knowles, 1990):

- Adults are motivated to learn as they experience needs and interests that learning will satisy; therefore, these are the appropriate starting points for organizing adult learning activities.
- Adults' orientation towards learning is life-centred; therefore, the appropriate units for organizing adult learning are life situations, not subjects.
- Experience is the richest resource for adults' learning; therefore, the core methodology of adult education is the analysis of experience.
- Adults have a deep need to be self-directing; therefore, the role of the teacher is to engage in a process of mutual inquiry with them rather than to transmit his or her knowledge to them and then evaluate their conformity to it.

- Individual differences among people increase with age; therefore, adult education must make optimal provision for differences of style, time, place and pace of learning (Knowles, 1990).

Knowles makes a distinction between **pedagogy** – or the theory and practice of the education of children and young people and **andragogy** – or the theory and practice of the education of adults. Knowles argues that adults differ from children in at least the following ways: biologically (in terms of their physical development), legally (in terms of what they are and are not allowed to do by law) and psychologically (in terms of the idea that adults are more able to take responsibility for their lives and be 'self-directed). Knowles then produces several assumptions that make up what he refers to as the 'andragogical model':

1. **The need to know**. Adults need to know why they need to learn something before undertaking to learn it.
2. **The learners' self-concept**. Adults have a self-concept of being responsible for their own decisions, for their own lives.
3. **The role of the learners' experience**. Adults come into an educational activity with both a greater volume and a different quality of experience from youths.
4. **Readiness to learn**. Adults become ready to learn those things they need to know and be able to do in order to cope effectively with their real-life situations.
5. **Orientation to learning**. In contrast to children's and youths' subject-centred orientation to learning (at least in school), adults are life-centred (or task centred or problem-centred) in their orientation to learning.
6. **Motivation**. While adults are responsive to some external motivators (better jobs, promotions, higher salaries...), the most potent motivators are internal pressures (the desire for increased job satisfaction, self-esteem, quality of life and the like) (Knowles, 1990).

Perhaps, we should be cautious. There is a danger of Knowles's generalizing too widely about the nature of adults. One might be tempted to suggest that many of his points apply more to employed adults, for example, than they do to those who are not working. Also, I suspect, a number of people in dull jobs are motivated more by external rewards than by internal motivation. However, despite these reservations (and the added one that many of the above principles may apply to children as well as to adults) the priniciples may be useful guidelines to helping to make decisions about professional education and training of the type described in this book. In many ways, the fundamental principles of andragogy echo the basic principles of experiential learning. Knowles suggests, for example, that self-concept, prior experience and the need to apply what you learn are all important in an adults' curriculum. All of these, as we have seen from Chapter 1, apply to the notion of experiential learning. They apply, too, to most health professionals in that most are caught up with the business of learning how to improve their interpersonal skills while, also, doing the job. Most health education training and education is not split off from practice (and most would argue, I suspect, that this is appropriate). Therefore, most trainees – and certainly most trained health care workers – are required to work in the field at the same time as learning **how** to work in the field.

Knowles and associates (1984) have identified seven components of andragogical practice that they feel are replicable in a variety of programmes and training workshops throughout the world. These components are highly relevant to the development of the experiential learning approach to interpersonal skills training:

- Facilitators must establish a physical and psychological climate conducive to learning. This is achieved physically by circular seating arrangements and psychologically by creating a climate of mutual respect among all participants, by emphasizing collaborative modes of learning, by establishing an atmosphere of mutual trust, by offering to be supportive and by emphasizing that learning is pleasant.
- Facilitators must involve learners in mutual planning of methods and curriculum directions. People will make firm commitments to activities in which they feel they have played a participatory, contributory role.
- Facilitators must involve themselves in diagnosing their own learning needs.
- Facilitators must encourage learners to formulate their own learning objectives.
- Facilitators must encourage learners to identify resources and to devise strategies for using such resources to accomplish their objectives.
- Facilitators must help learners to carry out their learning plans.
- Facilitators must involve learners in evaluating their learning, principally through the use of qualitative evaluation modes.

Out of this discussion on the philosophical underpinnings of two approaches to the curriculum arise certain practical considerations for programme planning for health educators wishing to plan interpersonal skills courses or workshops. Brookfield (1986) discusses what he calls the principles of practice in community action projects. These principles may well serve as the underlying principles for developing experiential learning workshops and training programmes for health care professionals and they underpin the principles described in this book in the discussion of experiential learning in a group setting:

- The medium of learning and action is the small group.
- Essential to the success of efforts is the development of collaborative solidarity among group members. This does not mean that dissension is silenced or divergence stifled; rather, group members are able to accept conflict, secure in the knowledge that their peers regard their continued presence in the group as vital to its success.
- The focus of the group's actions is determined after full discussion of participant's needs and full negotiation of all needs, including those of any formal 'educators' present.

- As adults undertake the actions they have collaboratively agreed upon, they develop an awareness of their collective power. This awareness is also felt when these adults renegotiate aspects of their personal, occupational and recreational lives.
- A successful initiative is one in which action and analysis alternate. Concentrating solely on action allows no time for the group to check its progress or alter previously agreed-upon objectives. But if the members of the group engage solely in analysis, they will never come to recognize their individuality and collective power. Empowerment is impossible without alternating action and reflection (Brookfield, 1986).

If Knowles and Brookfield are right, adults need to use what they learn. All interpersonal learning needs to be grounded in the participants' practical experience and any new learning needs to be the sort that can be applied on future occasions. Both Knowles's and Brookfield's notions of the educational principles of facilitating learning groups are entirely relevant to the running of interpersonal skills groups for health professionals in that all learners coming to such groups (regardless of their status and regardless of the specific discipline) are adults.

In order to demonstrate these principles in action it may be useful to consider an example of an experiential learning workshop in action.

ACQUIRING INTERPERSONAL SKILLS IN THE HEALTH PROFESSIONS: NUMBER 11

Critical incidents

Ask members of an interpersonal skills group to recall one of the following incidents:

- when you dealt with someone's emotional release ineffectually;
- when you dealt with someone's anger well;
- when you broke bad news to somebody and handled the situation adequately.

Then hold a discussion on what behaviours made those situations effective or not effective.

AN EXAMPLE OF AN EXPERIENTIAL WORKSHOP ON STRESS

It is useful to have some understanding of what an experiential learning workshop 'feels' like and how the philosophical issues discussed here can be translated into action. What follows is a description of the activities in a one-day workshop. It makes extensive use of the principles of experiential learning and adult learning described in this book and acknowledges some of the problems that may arise in this sort of workshop and which are discussed in more detail in the next chapter.

The workshop is attended by 18 health professionals from various disciplines including social work, nursing, occupational therapy and physiotherapy. The workshop is led by the author and takes place in a large room in a local higher education college. The group members are sat in a circle. Beside the facilitator is a large flip-chart pad on an easel. The workshop starts promptly at 9.00 pm.

The facilitator introduces himself and invites members of the group to introduce themselves by stating:

- their name,
- their occupation,
- three other things about themselves.

These three headings are revealed on a pre-prepared flip-chart sheet. The sheet with the headings is covered by a top sheet, which is turned over by the facilitator as he invites the group to introduce themselves.

Each member of the group then introduces themselves. Some take a little while over the task, others are faltering but fairly hasty. When each person has had a turn, the facilitator suggests that each person repeats, slowly, the name by which he or she wishes to be known. Thus the facilitator introduces himself by his first name. The round begins slowly but then speeds up and the facilitator urges the group to take time over the undertaking so that each person's name is heard by other members. This round is then followed by another slow name round. Group members are then invited to check the names of those people they are still unsure of. The facilitator checks one person's name and then others follow suit. The ice has been broken and the group looks and feels more relaxed.

Basic principles of the workshop are then spelt out. These are the voluntary principle, described above and the proposal clause, also described. The facilitator also spells out, clearly, the timing of the workshop, giving times of coffee, tea and lunch breaks. After this, he invites questions from the group. The group is clearly thawing out and beginning to talk more freely. A couple of people ask about the nature of the group and whether or not it will consist of lectures from the facilitator or not or whether or not it will be an 'encounter group'. The facilitator explains that the day will be activity-based and allow for participants to explore their own stress and stressors and examine some practical methods of dealing with stress. These questions lead naturally to the first exercise.

The exercise is carried out in pairs. Each pair nominates one member A and one B. A then talks to B for ten minutes about 'how I react to stress'. After ten minutes, A and B swop roles and B talks to A about his or her reactions to stress. The pair are asked to note that the exercise is not a conversation. One member is only required to listen while the other person talks. The exercise is a type of thinking out loud.

After the exercise, which has been timed by the facilitator (who, on this occasion is the odd man out in terms of numbers, so does not take part in the exercise), the pairs are invited back into the group. They then discuss the exercise in terms of **process** and **content**. Process refers to how it felt to do the exercise. Content refers to what was talked about.

The discussion is prolonged and thus forms the 'reflective' aspect of the experiential learning cycle. The facilitator could have written up the main points of the discussion, after it occurred, on one or more flip chart sheets but chose not to on this occasion. Such decisions are best taken in the heat of the moment. Sometimes the aide memoire is useful and the sheets can be pinned or 'bluetacked' up on the wall to serve as a backcloth to the workshop. On other occasions, the procedure seems to get in the way of the natural flow of the group's life.

Some of the issues that come up during the two aspects of the discussion are as follows:

- physical tension,
- loss of concentration,
- moodiness,
- lack of interest in work,
- difficulty with relationships,
- panic/fear,
- difficulty with sex,
- anxiety,
- frustration,
- feeling of being overwhelmed,
- loss of sleep,
- fatigue,
- depression,
- crying,
- walking away from the situation,
- going off sick,
- being judgemental of others,
- angry spells,
- etc.

The facilitator then asks the group for its reactions to the results of the discussion. Theories and comments put forward by group members include:

- 'We all seem to experience stress differently.'
- 'Some aspects of stress are common to all of us.'
- 'I thought I was the only one who got worked up over nothing: it's a relief!'

The discussion brings the first hour and a half to a close and the group breaks for coffee, still discussing the issues involved.

On resuming, after the break, the facilitator suggests that members divide into small groups of three and four and discuss some of the causes of stress, under three headings:

- How I cause myself stress
- How other people cause me stress
- Causes of stress within the world at large.

These headings are adapted from Bond's (1986) suggestions. Each group is given a flip chart sheet and a fibre-tipped pen and invited to elect a chairperson who writes down all the comments from the group. That chairperson does not edit out any suggestions but writes everything down. This is a typical brainstorming session. It is suggested that no filtering or dismissal of ideas takes place at all. In this way, the group develop freedom to think broadly and creatively. Some of the causes identified by group members are as follows:

How I cause myself stress

- by pushing myself too hard
- by having too greater expectations for myself
- by worrying too much
- by not being assertive
- by allowing other people to walk all over me
- by agreeing with everybody, even when I don't really!
- by thinking about sex too much
- by not getting what I want/need
- by suffering from loss of confidence/self-doubt
- by not thinking about my relationships with others
- by not planning my work
- by allowing myself to get depressed
- by allowing others to decide what I should do

How other people cause me stress

- by demanding too much of me
- by not agreeing with me
- by manipulating me
- by putting pressure on me to succeed
- by comparing me with other people (particularly at work)
- by not really knowing me
- by getting aggressive with me
- by belittling me.
- by being too bossy/authoritarian
- by not communicating with me
- by leaving me out in the cold
- by not being honest with me

- by being too easy with me
- by doing things I don't like
- by their anti-social habits (smoking, drinking etc.)

Causes of stress within the world at large

- violence and bombings
- child abuse
- 'pressure', in general
- lack of purpose
- speed
- rise in the cost of living
- rise in the mortgage rate
- abuse of animals
- lack of housing
- lack of health care resources
- unemployment
- the government

This exercise, in groups, runs for 20 minutes, after which time the facilitator invites group members to stick their charts up on the wall and to examine other people's charts as they go up. After this, there is a discussion about the process as well as the content of the exercise.

The group is invited to draw conclusions (or to theorize) about what has happened. Some responses, here, include:

- 'I mostly create my own stress!'
- 'I tend to believe that everyone is stressed for most of the time.'
- 'I'm suprised how quickly we have got to know each other here.'
- 'I found the discussion of sexuality embarrassing but useful.'

This exercise is the last of the morning. As a closing activity, each person in turn is asked to state, first of all, what they liked least about the morning. They are told that they need not qualify what they say but should feel free to say anything they like. After this round is completed, they are then encouraged to say what they liked most about the morning and again, it is suggested that they do not need to justify or qualify what they say. The facilitator joins in both rounds. Some of the comments from group members are illustrated below:

'What I liked least about the morning':

- the initial embarrassment;
- joining in with the pairs exercises, first thing;
- discussion of embarrassing subjects!;
- I thought things were a bit slow to start with.

'What I liked most about the morning':

- meeting new people;
- comparing experience with other people;
- realizing that other people feel the same as me!;
- pairing off;
- being listened to but not judged.

Before breaking for lunch, the facilitator proposes a brief 'unfinished business' session. In this period of five minutes, group members are invited to say anything they like, either to other group members or to the facilitator, either positive or negative, that they may be thinking or feeling. The rationale behind this activity (and this is made explicit to the group) is to raise any 'hidden agendas' and to allow further self-disclosure. It also works on the principle that it is perhaps better that things are said rather than just thought.

After an initial period of silence, one person says:

'I felt quite stirred up by the discussion this morning ... I'm surprised how easily I get worked up ...'

Another says:

'I'm a bit annoyed that you rushed me this morning (to the facilitator) and would have preferred more time to finish what I was saying!'

One member says to another:

'I enjoyed the pairs exercise with you this morning. I think we've got quite a bit in common!'

After the five minutes, the group disperses and goes to lunch.

The afternoon session starts with a modified 'icebreaker'. Each person is invited to say something about themselves that they are proud of. It may be something that they have achieved or a personal quality. As usual, the facilitator takes part in the round. The round seems to recreate an atmosphere in which group members can easily talk and self-disclose.

Following this, the group brainstorms methods of relieving stress. In this activity, the facilitator acts as scribe and records the suggestions of the group on a series of flip-chart sheets. Examples of some of the methods of stress relief that are identified by the group include the following:

- sleep
- walking/cycling/exercise
- massage
- drinking alcohol
- using tranquillizers in small doses
- having a bath
- eating
- smoking

- relaxation exercises
- time management
- taking sick leave
- taking a holiday
- meditation
- yoga
- having a good laugh/cry
- counselling and co-counselling
- change of activity
- organization
- discussion of relationships with the people involved
- learning to be assertive
- etc.

A discussion is then developed on the most common methods of stress relief, the ones that work and the ones that don't. As with the morning's session, there is some surprise and some relief that many people's experiences are similar.

The facilitator then asks the group to choose two methods from the list with which they are not particularly familiar and which they would like to try. After a brief discussion, they choose meditation and relaxation exercises. The facilitator then gives a brief theory input on the nature of relaxation exercises and on meditation. Theoretical information for such inputs can be found in Naranjo and Ornstein (1971); Hewitt (1977); Bond (1986); Bond and Kilty (1986).

After this, the group undertakes a relaxation exercise. Once the relaxation activity has been undertaken, the group reforms and discusses the process of the activity. All but one member has experienced complete relaxation. The one person has found that, paradoxically, she feels more tense through undertaking the activity and this is talked through with the person, with the group's support. After the discussion of her feelings, she feels considerably relieved and realizes that she gets most relief from stress through talking about the stressors in her life. This is useful both for her and for a number of other group members.

Following this discussion, the facilitator leads the group in a short meditation. The procedure for this is as follows:

1. Sit motionless, comfortably and with the eyes closed.
2. Breathe quietly and gently. Breathe in through the nostrils and out through the mouth.
3. Let your attention focus on your breathing,
4. Begin to count your breaths, from one to ten. One is the whole cycle of inhalation and exhalation. Two is the next complete cycle.
5. When the breaths have been counted from one to ten, begin counting the next ten and then the next and so on.

6. If you are distracted or lose count, simply return to the beginning of the process and start again.

Following the 15 minute meditation, the group are again invited to discuss what happened. This time, all members find the activity relaxing and de-stressing and remarks are made about how they were physically and mentally able to relax. A member requests details of the two activities and the facilitator offers pre-prepared handouts of them (the two described in this book may be freely used by other health professionals who wish to use them for handout purposes as long as acknowledgment of source is given). Many say that they wish to carry on using either the relaxation script or the meditation, at other times, away from the workshop.

After tea, there is an open-ended discussion about the day's events. Participants are invited to identify the high and low spots of the day and a closing round of 'least liked' and 'most liked' is carried out. The workshop finishes on a calm but interested note and group members feel that it has been an interesting and worthwhile workshop.

The workshop described here is just one example of how the experiential learning cycle may be put into practice. Not all the suggestions and principles suggested by Knowles and Brookfield are present in the example but a number are and the general principles of experiential and adult learning may be noted. It will also be noted that plenty of time was allowed for discussing each activity and that there was very little theory input into the day. This is in keeping with the notion of moving away from the facilitator occupying a teaching role towards a more facilitative role, as described above.

THE NEED FOR LIFELONG EDUCATION

More than anything else, no sort of educational or training enterprise should be viewed as a conclusive process. All learning is provisional and everything we learn should be open to question – including the skills that we learn. A few moments' reflection will reveal that interpersonal skills, like other sorts, go in and out of fashion. What was the appropriate way of answering the telephone a few years ago has been overtaken by a much more 'professional' way. How we expect medical consultants to act has changed radically – we expect them to offer a much more 'human' face than may have been the case a few decades ago. All of this underpins the need for us to invest in **lifelong** education. Malcolm Knowles suggests that the need for lifelong education is based on the following assumptions:

1. Learning in a world of acceleration change must be a lifelong process.
2. Learning is a process of active inquiry with the initiative residing in the learner.

3. The purpose of education is to facilitate the development of the competencies required for performance in life situations.
4. Learners are highly diverse in their experiential backgrounds, pace of learning, readiness to learn, and styles of learning; therefore, learning programmes need to be highly individualized.
5. Resources for learning abound in every environment; a primary task of a learning system is to identify these resources and link learners with them effectively.
6. People who have been taught in traditional schools have on the whole been conditioned to perceive the proper role of learners as being dependent on teachers to make decisions for them as to what should be learned, how it should be learned, when it should be learned, and if it has to be learned; they therefore need to be helped to make the transition to becoming self-directed learners.
7. Learning (even self-directed learning) is enhanced by interaction with others.
8. Learning is more efficient if guided by a process of structure (e.g. learning plan) than by a content structure (e.g. course outline) (Knowles, 1990).

Knowles, here, again emphasizes a focus on individualized learning. In a sense, of course, we all become 'individualized learners' once we finish formal education or training programs. Most of us, as working professionals, continue to read journals and books, attend study days or conferences and talk to each other about issues concerning the profession. However, we also probably need to do more than this. Many professional health care bodies are now making further education mandatory as part of the professional's process of re-registering as a practitioner. In the future it seems likely that most health care professionals will have to offer evidence of having undertaken further education throughout their careers. And all of this seems completely in line with the suggestions that Knowles is making, above – accept, of course, that the process is no longer a chosen one but a prescribed one. It remains to be seen the degree to which forcing people to accept further training and education will make them better practitioners. It seems likely, though, that as the process of continual updating becomes the norm for any given profession, the professionals within it will come to see this updating as appropriate and inevitable. In an ideal world, perhaps, people would choose to update. As things stand, it seems likely that many professionals need a bit of a shove to make them move in the direction of updating – a point that seems to work against Knowles's idea that most adults are driven, necessarily, by internal motivators.

In the next chapter, the focus of the discussion shifts from general principles to specific examples of facilitation. Through considering her underlying educational beliefs and values and through considering the specific skills of facilitation, the health professional who teaches interpersonal skills can enhance and develop her ability and effectiveness.

6

Facilitating learning groups

FACILITATION OR TEACHING?

As we noted in the previous chapter, the accent in the experiential learning approach is towards the educational encounter being student-centred rather than teacher centred and appropriately adult-centred. In this approach, the aim is not to initiate the group participants into particular ways of knowing, as Peters (1969) would argue, but to encourage those people to think about their own experience and to transform their personal knowledge and skills through the processes of reflection, discussion and action.

John Heron (1989) defines facilitation in the following way:

> What I mean by a facilitator ... is a person who has the role of helping participants to learn in an experiential group. The facilitator will normally be formally appointed to this role by whatever organization is sponsoring the group. And the group members will voluntarily accept the facilitator in this role (Heron, 1989).

Elizabeth King offers the following suggestions about the nature of the facilitator's role:

- They must believe students should make their own decisions and think for themselves.
- They must refrain from assuming an authoritative role and adopt a more facilitative and listening position.
- They must accept diversity of race, sex, values etc, among their students.
- They must be willing to accept all viewpoints unconditionally and not impose their personal values on the students. The ability to entertain alternatives and to negotiate no-lose solutions to problems often leads to group decisions that are more beneficial for both the individual and the group.

Hovand and his colleagues (Hovand et al., 1953; Hovand and Janis, 1959; Rosenberg and Hovand, 1960) undertook research into which kind of facilitator styles were most likely to have an impact on a group. They identified the importance of credibility in the success of a leader in an experiential workshop. They suggest that credibility consists of:

1. the ability to communicate a sense of competence in relation to the topic which provides the focus for the workshop activity – this competence can derive either from scholarship or experience or some combination of both;
2. being perceived as reliable as far as information sources are concerned – the extent to which workshop participants feel that the leader is dependable, predictable and consistent;
3. having one's motives clearly understood, especially in situations of conflict or when risks are being taken by participants;
4. being empathetic, warm and genuine in one's relations with participants;
5. the degree of dynamism or charisma displayed by the leader – indicated by the control and activity-leadership displayed and the extent to which participants feel confident about the direction offered by the leader; and
6. majority opinion of the group – pressure towards conformity in workshops is high.

Janis (1982) drew up a check-list of features of helping which maximized the helpers' ability to influence those with thom they worked. Here are some of the skills that he regards as critical:

- encouraging participants to make self-disclosures;
- giving positive feedback to participants and showing both acceptance and understanding of their feelings and thoughts;
- using helping skills to reshape thoughts presented by participants so as to encourage them to develop fresh insights;
- being concrete – making direct statements which endorse practical suggestions made by participants and which give direction to some workshop or helping activity;
- eliciting commitment to taking some action (for example, to read more, to discuss with a colleague some aspect of the workshop and so on) – encouraging participants to develop a self-contract for work as a result of the workshop process;
- showing that the ideas expressed by group members have antecedents in the work of other people – connecting 'naive' ideas to bodies of research and/or theory;
- giving selective positive feedback so as to shape the direction of an individual's development during a workshop;
- undertaking direct training of a person or sub-group or group so as to give some practical skills;
- giving reassurances to individuals within the group that they are learning and developing;
- being explicit about the contract for the workshop and its termination;

- giving reminders as to the major features of learning that have occurred during the workshop; and
- building up the confidence of participants so that they can take some of the learning that has occurred during the workshop and apply it to situations that they encounter in the 'real' world (Janis, 1982).

Woolfe suggests, among other things, the following principles for undertaking the role of trainer in experiential workshops:

- Control of the nature and content of learning is shifted away from the trainer towards the student.
- The trainer has to allow students to make mistakes.
- Groups need structure, but in experiential learning many boundaries may have to be negotiated with the participants.
- The trainer has to be prepared to become redundant. This may involve learning how to cope with feelings of being unwanted.
- Sometimes groups coalesce and form an identity through the process of identifying an outside, against whom they can react. This outsider is frequently the facilitative leader. The trainer has be able to work through this process and to be sufficiently self-aware to acknowledge that the rejection may have more to do with the needs of the group members than with any personal inadequacies in himself or herself (Woolfe, 1992).

The last point is particularly interesting as Woolfe is beginning to hint at some of the **processes** that can occur when experiential groups are facilitated. More information about group processes is offered later in this chapter. Suffice to note, at this point, perhaps, is that the idea of **facilitation** is very different to that of teaching. Some of those diferences have been described in earlier chapters but a summary of them may be offered as follows:

1. In **facilitation** there is an accent on what the **learner** wants and needs rather than on working to a pre-set syllabus or programme.
2. In **facilitation**, the group leader offers a more **personal** teaching style both by role modelling and by encouraging students to disclose their own feelings and share their own experiences.
3. In **facilitation**, attention is paid to **group process** – what happens during the group sessions as well as what is **learned** during those sessions.
4. In **facilitation**, the group leader works more as an **equal** with other group members and does not assume that he or she is necessarily cleverer or better informed than other group members.
5. In **facilitation** there is structure, but that structure is determined by the needs of everyone in the group and not just determined by the group leader.
6. In **facilitation**, much attention is paid to an individual's ability to monitor themselves and to self-assess.

Certain stages in the facilitation process can be described and the facilitator needs to be aware of the processes that can occur in groups. The stages described here are modified from those offered by Malcolm Knowles (1975) in his discussion of facilitating learning groups for adults.

It is arguable that facilitation of learning has more in common with group therapy than it does with teaching. It is recommended that the person who sets out to become a group facilitator gain experience as a member of a number of different sorts of groups before leading one herself. In this way she will not only learn about group processes experientially but she will also see a number of facilitator styles. As Heron (1977b) points out, in the early stages of becoming a facilitator, it is often helpful to base your style on a facilitator that you have seen in action. Later, the style becomes modified in the light of your own experience and you develop your own approach.

ACQUIRING INTERPERSONAL SKILLS IN THE HEALTH PROFESSIONS: NUMBER 12

Giving feedback about change

In an interpersonal skills group that is composed of members that trust each other, try a 'round' whereby each person sits and receives comments about what other members of the group would like to change about that person. The exercise can be a good one for developing the skills of giving negative feedback tactfully and carefully.

This exercise needs to be managed carefully. The aim is not to be 'negative' for its own sake but to encourage the development of skills in tactfully helping other people to change through feedback. The facilitator should watch, carefully, for tactless or hurtful comments and, if possible 'intercept' them and rule them out. This sort of 'monitoring' by the facilitator (although it involves a degree of personal judgement) is yet another way of role-modelling constructive feedback.

STAGES IN THE FACILITATION PROCESS

Setting the learning climate

The first aspect of helping adults to learn is the creation of an atmosphere in which adult learners feel comfortable and thus able to learn. This is particularly important when it comes to developing interpersonal skills through experiential learning. Unlike more formal classroom learning, the experiential approach asks of the learners that they try things out, take some risks and experiment. If this is to happen at all, it needs to be undertaken in an atmosphere of mutual trust and understanding.

The first aspect of the setting of a learning climate is to ensure that the environment is appropriate. Rows of desks and chairs are reminiscent of earlier schooldays. For the adult experiential learning group it is often better and certainly more egalitarian if learners and facilitator sit together in a closed circle of chairs. Experiential learning workshops rarely involve a great deal of note taking, so desks or tables rarely serve as anything more than a barrier between learners and facilitator.

In the early stages of a workshop or learning group it is useful if the group members spend time getting to know each other. 'Icebreakers' are sometimes used for this purpose. An icebreaker is a simple group activity that is designed to relax people and allow them to 'let their hair down' a little, thus creating a more relaxed atmosphere, arguably more conducive to learning interpersonal skills. Three examples of icebreakers are as follows.

Icebreaker 1

The group stands up and group members mill around the room at will. At a signal from the facilitator, each person stops and introduces herself to the nearest person and share some personal details. Then each person moves on and, at a further signal, stop and greet another person in a similar way. This series of millings and pairings can continue until each group member has met every other, including the facilitator.

Icebreaker 2

A small cushion is used in this icebreaker. After each person in the group, in turn, has introduced herself, by name, the cushion is thrown by the facilitator to one group member. As it is thrown, the facilitator calls out the name of the person who is receiving the cushion. That person then throws the cushion to another person and calls out that person's name. This activity carries on until all members of the group have learned the names of people in the group. The activity is a lighthearted affair and one that encourages the learning of member's names through repetition ... identifying needs.

Icebreaker 3

The group splits into pairs for five minutes. During that five minutes, each member of the pairs 'interviews' the other and finds out five or six things about them (including their name). After the five minutes, the group reforms and each person introduces the person that they spoke with.

Other examples of icebreaking activities can be found elsewhere (Heron, 1973; Brandes and Phillips, 1984; Burnard, 1985). Their aim is to produce a relaxed atmosphere in which learning can take place and a further gain is that they encourage group participation and the learning of names. They are used by many facilitators in the experiential learning field. Some people, however (including the author) feel more comfortable with a more straightforward form of introduction. The argument, here, is that learners coming to a new learning experience are already apprehensive. Many carry with them memories of past learning experiences that may or may not have been of the 'formal' sort. To introduce those people to icebreakers too early may be to alienate them before they start. The icebreaker, by its very unorthodoxy, may surprise and upset them. A simpler form of introductory activity is to invite each person in turn to tell the rest of the group the following information:

- their name;
- where they work and their position in the team or organization;
- a few details about themselves that are nothing to do with work.

It is helpful if the facilitator sets the pace for the activity by first introducing herself in this way. A precedent is thus set and the group members have some idea of both what to say and how much to say. The author recalls forgetting this principle when running a workshop in the Netherlands. As a result, each group member talked for about ten minutes apiece and what was intended to be a short introductory activity turned into a lengthy exercise! The golden rule, perhaps, is to keep the activity short and sharp and keep the atmosphere 'light' and easy-going.

Once group members have begun to get to know each other, either through the use of icebreakers or by the introductory activity described above, the facilitator should deal with 'domestic' issues regarding the group's life. These will include the following:

- when the group will break for refreshments and meal breaks and when it will end;
- a discussion of the aims of the group;
- a discussion of the 'voluntary principle': that learners should decide for themselves whether or not they will take place in any given activity suggested by the facilitator and that no one should feel pressurized into taking part in any activity either by the facilitator or by the power of group pressure; it is worth pointing out that if a person finds themselves to be the only person sitting out on a particular activity, they should not feel under any further obligation either (a) to take part or (b) to justify their decision not to take part;
- issues relating to smoking in the group, when smokers are present;
- any other issues identified by either the facilitator or by group members.

This early discussion of group 'rules' is an important part of the process of setting the learning climate. The structure engendered by this part of the day helps to allow everyone to feel part of the decision making and learning process.

Identifying learning resources

Most interpersonal skills workshops run for people in the caring professions are attended by adults who have considerable life experience and work skills. They have always had considerable learning experience prior to attending such a workshop. The aim of the next stage of group development is to identify skills within the group that may serve as resources for further learning. Examples of such skills, that may be used as examples of learning models for others may include such things as:

- specific counselling skills;
- skills with particular client groups, e.g. the elderly, adolescents, people with AIDS, etc.;
- previous experience in groups;
- etc.

Once such skills have been identified, they can be made use of by the group as and when opportunities arise. They can also be more formally 'written in' to the aims of the learning group by setting aside time for those people with skills to demonstrate them or through their facilitating teaching sessions with the rest of the group. It is at this stage that the facilitator needs to retain some humility. It is often difficult to appreciate, when you are running a group, that other people in that group may be more skilled than you in various respects!

Running the learning group

All that remains, once the learning climate has been established and resources within the group have been identified, is for the facilitator to establish the smooth running of the group throughout the use of various activities aimed at enhancing learning. In the last chapter of this book, a variety of exercises is offered as examples of the sorts of group activities that can be used to encourage the learning of specific interpersonal skills. Following the pattern laid down by the experiential learning cycle discussed earlier, these stages may be used in this part of the workshop:

1. brief theory input;
2. description of the exercise to be undertaken;
3. setting up of the activity with group members;
4. running of the activity;
5. discussion of group members' experiences following the activity.

Thus, for example, the first part of a workshop on counselling skills may be prefaced by a short theory input by the facilitator or by another member of the group, on the subject of listening. This input need not be a lecture but is often best treated as a fairly informal discussion, drawing on group member's experiences. Following this theory input, an exercise taken from the last chapter of this book is described to the group and instructions given as to pairing, timing and so on. The group then does the exercise. After this, two options present themselves for 'processing' the outcome of the exercise. Group members may either:

(a) stay in their pairs and discuss the activity, before returning to a larger plenary session with the rest of the group, or

(b) return to the group for a discussion led by the facilitator.

Whichever format is used, the facilitator may choose to discuss either the **process** of the activity or the **content** of it. The process of an activity refers to what it felt like to undertake that activity and what learning followed as a result of those feelings. A discussion of the content is one that discusses what was talked about. In interpersonal skills training, it may be more productive to spend more time discussing the process of any given exercise than the content. In this way, group members develop the skill of noticing their own behaviour in interpersonal situations. Indeed, it is sometimes helpful to suggest that the content of pairs and small group activities remains confidential to those people taking part in the activity and that such content does not become part of the general discussion of the group. In this way, the group can quickly learn to handle true selfdisclosure in a safe atmosphere: a situation that closely resembles many 'real-life' interpersonal encounters that the health professional will have to face.

It is useful to spend considerable time in this post-exercise discussion. Referring back to the experiential learning cycle discussed in a previous chapter, it was noted that Kolb (1984) asserts that new learning occurs when people reflect on their behaviour. The discussion following an exercise is an example of such reflection and the reflective process takes time. It should not be rushed by the facilitator nor should she attempt to suggest what outcomes the group members may have discovered through doing the exercise. It is common, in more traditional educational settings for a teacher to ask questions that begin:

'Did you notice how ...?'

or

'Most people find ... when they do this sort of exercise'.

Such questions have little relevance in this sort of educational experience. The aim is not to lead the group participants in a particular direction but to enable them to undertake the reflective process themselves and decide, for themselves, whether or not they will share their experience with other people. More useful questions, from a facilitation point of view, would be:

'What did you notice ...?'

or

'Does anyone want to talk about what they experienced during that exercise ...?'

'What else happened ...?'

This is true 'facilitation' as opposed to 'teaching'. This aspect of experiential learning also points up a particular paradox. While the facilitator will be aiming to encourage the development of counselling, assertiveness or group skills, there is no guarantee that all group members will develop the same sorts of skills nor even that they will develop the ones that the facilitator had in mind! It is quite possible that, through the process of experiential learning, certain group members find 'different' ways of dealing with aspects of counselling or group work, that had not occurred to the facilitator or that is not written up in the literature. This, perhaps, is the creative aspect of experiential learning and is in contrast to the usual type of learning that involves the passing on of previously established knowledge or skills.

Closing the group

Each facilitator will probably develop her own style of closing the group at the end of the day or at the end of a workshop. A traditional way is through summary of what the day has been about. There is an important limitation in this method, which aims at 'closure'. It is asserted that while the facilitator is summing up in this way, she is doing two things that are not particularly helpful. First, she is putting into her own words, those of the group members. Second, while she is 'closing' in this way, group members are often, silently, closing off their thoughts about the day or the workshop in much the same way that schoolchildren begin to put their books away as soon as a teacher sums up at the end of a lesson. It may be far better to leave the session open-ended and to avoid any sort of summing up. Alternatively, rather than allowing the day or the workshop to end rather abruptly, the facilitator may choose to use one or more of the following closing and evaluating activities:

Closing activity 1

Each person in turn makes a short statement about what they liked least about the day or about the workshop. Each person in turn then makes a short statement about what they liked most about the day or the workshop. No one has to justify what they say for their statement is taken as a personal evaluation of their feelings and experience.

Closing activity 2

Each person in turn makes a short statement about three things that they feel they have learned during the day or the workshop. This may or may not be followed by a discussion on the day's learning.

Closing activity 3

The group has an 'unfinished business' session. Group members are encouraged to share any comments they may have about the day or the workshop, either of a positive or negative nature. The rationale for this activity is that such sharing helps to avoid bottled-up feelings and increases a sense of group cohesion.

Closing activity 4

The group hug. Group members stand in a circle and put their arms around each others shoulders, to form a tightly knit circle. The group remains silent throughout this group exercise and agreement is made that people may be free to share any comments they may have with the group. This sort of symbolic activity may be particularly useful when self-disclosure has been high and people are feeling rather sensitive. It can help to encourage group cohesion, support and unity. Like all activities, however, it should not be a compulsory exercise: some people are naturally uncomfortable with an activity of this sort and the wise facilitator will chose this sort of activity with care!

These, then, are the stages of a typical interpersonal skills workshop and they may be adapted to suit the particular needs of the group and of the facilitator. The reader may like to refer back to the previous chapter to the example of a typical workshop and see to what degree the example there follows the stages described above.

GROUP DYNAMICS AND PROCESSES

Tuckman (1965) summarized the results of more than 50 studies into group development and formulated the following model of group development:

Stage 1: forming, characterized by testing and dependence;
Stage 2: storming, characterized by intragroup conflict;
Stage 3: norming, characterized by the development of group cohesion; and
Stage 4: performing, characterized by the group working as a team.

Fay and Doyle (1992) offered the following description of the main features of each stage of the Tuckman model.

Stage 1: forming

- attempts to identify tasks in terms of relevant parameters and to decide how the group will accomplish the tasks
- decisions on the type of information needed and how it will be used
- hesitant participation
- test of behavioural expectations and ways to handle behavioural problems
- feelings of initial attachment to the team
- intellectualizing
- discussion of symptoms or problems peripheral to the task
- complaints about the organizational environment
- suspicion, fear, and anxiety about the new situation
- minimal work accomplishment

Stage 2: storming

- infighting, defensiveness and competition
- establishment of unachievable goals
- disunity, increased tension and jealousy
- resistance to the task demands because they are perceived to interfere with personal needs
- polarization of group members
- sharp fluctuations of relationships and reversals of feelings
- concern over excessive work
- establishment of pecking orders
- minimal work accomplishment

Stage 3: norming

- an attempt to achieve maximum harmony by avoiding conflict
- a high level of intimacy characterized by confiding in each other, sharing personal problems and discussing team dynamics
- a new ability to express emotions constructively
- a sense of team cohesiveness with a common spirit and goals
- the establishment and maintenance of team boundaries
- moderate work accomplishment

Stage 4: performing

- members experience insights into personal and interpersonal processes
- constructive self-change is undertaken
- a great deal of work is accomplished (Fay and Doyle, 1992).

Apart from considering the stages of group facilitation and development that are involved in planning a group learning session or a workshop, the facilitator also needs to know something about the dynamics or processes that can occur in such a group. The idea, here, is that to be forewarned is to be forearmed! In this section, some of those processes are described and suggestions offered as to how those processes can be coped with as they occur. In the end, there can be no one way of coping with a particular process: everything is dependent upon the people concerned, the context, the perceptions of the facilitator and of group members and so on.

Pairing

Pairing in groups refers to one or other of two phenomena. First, the word can refer to two group members who talk quietly to each other, ignoring the rest of the group. It is arguable that such a manoeuvre is a defensive one in that the pair are avoiding issues being discussed in the larger group by talking to each other.

Pairing of this sort can be distracting to the facilitator and disruptive to the group because it means that the group is not operating as a single unit but is divided.

The second type of pairing is when two group members (and one is sometimes the facilitator) tend to discuss issues with each other, across the group, rather than sharing a 'whole group' discussion. This sort of pairing is less distracting than the previous sort but can cause problems. If the facilitator consistently pairs with another person in the group, that facilitator may tend to ignore other group members.

A variety of options are available to the facilitator for dealing with pairing when it occurs. Some of these are:

- ignore it and see what happens; sometimes, pairing takes care of itself;
- draw attention to the fact that pairing has occurred and allow the group to resolve the issue;
- confront the two persons concerned; this must be done carefully if it is not to cause reminders of schooldays and bossy teachers!;
- suggest that the group members all change seats as an 'icebreaking' activity;
- set a contract with the group, prior to the group's development, that all members will be on the lookout for the occurrence of such dynamics;
- engage one of the pair in discussion so that the pairing is at least temporarily broken up.

Scapegoating

Scapegoating is a name for the situation where one person in the group becomes the one who the group attacks, for whatever reason. Sometimes only one or two people are involved in the attack, sometimes everyone is involved. Again, it is arguable that this is a defensive manoeuvre in that the scapegoated person becomes a focal point for the pent-up aggression of the collective group. Sometimes, the person singled out for scapegoating is a particularly strong person who is well able to cope with the hostility. At other times, a weaker member becomes the focus. The facilitator has at least the following options when scapegoating occurs.

- Stop it. This is particularly important when a weaker member of the group is under attack.
- Draw attention to its happening and allow the group to deal with it.
- Suggest a short break in the group's activities.
- Switch the discussion suddenly to another topic so as to reduce tension. This can usually only be a temporary measure.
- Ask the scapegoated person how he is feeling about what is happening and take the cue for what to do from him.

Projecting

Projection, in a group context, is where one or more of the group members identifies a mood or a quality in the group that is, in fact, a mood of a quality of that
person. For example, a group member who is projecting his own anxiety may
say 'I find this a very tense group', when all the other group members feel
relaxed. It is clearly important to distinguish between descriptive comments
about the group and examples of projections! Sometimes a group member will
be offering a useful description of what is happening in the group and this
should not be too readily written off as projection.

Another version of projection is when the group-as-a-whole comes to view
an aspect of the world-outside-the-group in a hostile or aggressive way. For
example, common group projection is the 'group moan', where members get
caught up in a fairly circular discussion about how dreadful the 'organization'
or 'management' is and how helpless the group is given these circumstances.
Again, it is important for the facilitator to be able to distinguish between the
group describing an accurate situation and a group projection.

When projection occurs, the facilitator can try one or more of the following
interventions:

- ignore it and see what happens;
- offer the idea of projection to the group as a group 'interpretation' and see
  what the group does with the idea;
- ask the group to consider what they think may be happening in the group and
  allow it to make its own interpretations.

'League of Gentlemen'

This expression was coined by John Heron (1973) and refers to a variant of
pairing, whereby a small subgroup of people disrupt a group by forming a
hostile and often sarcastic body of people whose aim is to make life in the group
difficult. Often such a league is formed by one central and dominant figure who
draws into quiet discussion, by use of sub-vocal 'asides', the members of the
group sitting either side of him. It is recommended that the league of gentlemen
is always dealt with fairly quickly, for otherwise its effects can be very detri-
mental to the life of the group. Confronting the league of gentlemen is nearly
always difficult. Some suggestions of how this can be achieved include the
following.

- Direct confrontation: the subgroup leader is challenged about what is happening. This nearly always leads to a power struggle between the facilitator and
  the leader of the 'league of gentlemen'.
- The facilitator asks the group to notice what is happening in the group and
  allows the 'league of gentlemen' to surface as an issue. Unfortunately, it may
  not!

- The facilitator discloses her own discomfort at what is happening within the group. This intervention is often disarming to the league.

Wrecking

This is a 'one-person' version of the league of gentlemen. Here, an individual member of the group, for whatever reason, attempts to sabotage the group. This can take place in a variety of ways. The person may, for instance, consistently disagree with everything the facilitator says or does. He may refuse to take part in any activities and encourage others to do the same. He may always be late in coming to the group or suddenly walk out of it. He may, on the other hand, offer non-verbal resistance by remaining silent but indicating constant displeasure by use of facial expression. Wrecking as a group process often occurs when people are 'sent' to interpersonal skills training groups rather than coming of their own volition. A number of interventions are available:

- The person may be directly confronted about his behaviour. As with direct confrontation of the league of gentlemen, the confrontation is likely to be met with direct denial and a power struggle ensue between the wrecker and the facilitator.
- The group's attention may be drawn to the fact that something is happening within the group and comments invited.
- The facilitator may choose to talk to the person, on his own, outside of the group and try to reach an understanding of what is happening. Sometimes, wrecking behaviour can be a cover for deep unhappiness or distress on the part of the wrecker. Whether or not the facilitator chooses to investigate the deeper meanings of the wrecking behaviour will depend on the facilitator's beliefs about the aims of the group and on her expertise and training in that sort of work.

Flight

Sometimes the intensity of a group becomes too much for an individual member of the entire group. Emotions have been stirred, people are feeling threatened, it seems likely that someone will openly express emotion. At such times, it is not uncommon for the individual or the group to 'take flight'. They do this by changing the subject, injecting humour into the discussion, or by becoming silent. If the facilitator is unaware of what is happening, she may find that she, too, has taken flight, and the discussion has quickly moved away from its original subject.

There are various ways of handling flight, including the following.

- Point out to the group that it is happening and allow the group to take its own course.

- Ignore it and see what happens.
- Encourage it. This is to work paradoxically (Riebel, 1984). The paradoxical intervention is one that is apparently the completely wrong intervention at the right time. Thus, by encouraging the behaviour that is happening is to take a step towards changing that behaviour. An example from a therapeutic context may help here. The normal response to someone who is suffering from extreme anxiety is to help them to calm down. They may be asked to take deep breaths or to try to relax. Yet these are the very things that they cannot do! The paradoxical approach is to suggest that they become even more anxious. Very frequently, when a person is encouraged (or 'allowed') to do this, they laugh and find the anxiety beginning to drain away. Arguably what has happened is that they have been encouraged and allowed to do the very thing that they are good at doing. In the process, they have found the means to reverse their problem. So it is with encouraging flight in a group. As the group is encouraged to change tack or to laugh so they quickly come to acknowledge what they have been doing. It is usually not long before someone in the group picks up the fact that the group has been running away from itself. The paradoxical approach to working with groups and interpersonal skills training workshops is an interesting and varied one. The method of encouraging a group activity that you want to change is always an option (Heron, 1986; Fay, 1978).
- Gently bring the group or the individual back on track and away from the flight. After this has happened, it is useful to go back and discuss what has happened.

Shutting down

This is a particular sort of internal flight that can occur when an individual in a group is threatened by what is happening in that group. When a person shuts down, they become silent and withdrawn and appear to be taking little interest in what is going on in the group. Shutting down usually only occurs in groups where emotions are running high or where 'hidden agenda' (see below) have been suddenly made explicit. The shut-down person needs gentle handling and some of the options are as follows.

- Offering simple, physical support, if the person is sitting next to the facilitator. If the facilitator reaches out and merely touches the person or holds their hand or arm, it can help the person to feel acknowledged. It may also trigger off the release of pent-up emotion and the person may begin to cry. In this case it is often helpful if the facilitator can allow the emotion and thus enable the shut down person to gently 'thaw out'.
- Acknowledging, verbally, that the facilitator is aware of the shut-down person. Here, the facilitator allows the person to express some of the things that they are feeling. Again, pent-up emotion may be expressed.

- Moving on to new topics. If the shut-down person is finding the group heavy-going, it is sometimes kinder to change the subject that is under discussion to a more emotionally neutral one. Arguably, however, this is merely to put off the time when the issues that have caused the person to become shut down, are discussed.
- Asking the group to support the shut-down person. Here, the group is made aware that one of its members is cutting himself off from the group's activities and the group is asked for suggestions for helping that person. This intervention, if it is used badly, can slip rapidly into group patronage!

Rescuing

Rescuing is the opposite of scapegoating. Here, a member of the group is always being protected by one or more other members of the group. Sometimes, the person being rescued sets themselves up to be rescued. They may, for example, offer to the group a presentation of self that says, 'I can't cope and need help.' Clearly, too, a degree of rescuing is reasonable in that we all need to be helped out sometimes when the going gets rough. On the other hand, persistent rescuing disallows the person being rescued the chance to make decisions for himself or to find ways of coping with difficult situations within the group. In the health care professions, there are often a number of people who are 'compulsive carers' and who always want everything to work out well. When a group contains a number of such people, it is usually inevitable that considerable rescuing will take place. The facilitator can use at least one or more of the following interventions when rescuing occurs:

- ignore it and see what happens,
- ask the person being rescued what he would like to do,
- confront the rescuer directly,
- consult the group about what they think is going on in the group,
- ask the person being rescued to speak for himself.

Hidden agenda

In all groups, at least two things are happening: the group is following an overt or obvious agenda – the activities that they are engaged in. At another level, however, all sorts of hidden or undisclosed 'agenda' are being played out. These are the issues and problems that group members bring to the group that lay outside of the main or overt agenda. Kilty (1987) makes a useful set of distinctions between three sorts of hidden agenda that are frequently at work in an interpersonal skills learning group: work agenda, interpersonal agenda and personal agenda. Work agenda are those concerned with perceived competence and relationships at work. The person who is hiding an agenda about work may be thinking, as they sit in the group, 'What do my colleagues think of my performance so far?' or 'Have I damaged my reputation at work?'

Interpersonal agenda are concerned with rivalries, competition, conflicts and so forth. The person who is working from an interpersonal hidden agenda may be wondering 'Does the group leader still like me?' or 'Do people in this group think themselves more intelligent than me?' and so forth. Personal agenda are to do with the individual's own concerns about themselves and their lives. The person who is working with a personal agenda may be wondering, 'Can I cope with the emotional intensity of this group?' or 'Will I get very upset if I take part in this role play ... and then, what will happen?'

Hidden agendas affect the life of the group in that issues from such agenda are 'playing in the background' of the life of the group at all times. Sometimes, too, they emerge and become part of the regular or overt agenda. For example, when two group members disagree in a group discussion, the hidden agenda may emerge when one says to the other, 'That's typical ... you always thought you were better than me, anyway ... you're always like that at work!' Here, the issue is no longer confined to what is happening in the group but has become an issue of personal disagreement and disharmony that may have been simmering in the background for days, months or years and has suddenly become explicit. When hidden agenda become overt in this way, the facilitator has at least two options.

- To allow the hidden agenda issue to play itself out between the members of the group. This is the 'softer' option and may be useful when there is neither time nor a contract with the group to explore personal issues.
- To invite the group to explore the hidden agenda that is emerging. This is the more confronting option. It needs to be handled tactfully and non-judgementally by the facilitator and by the rest of the group and is probably more appropriate to a mature group (either in terms of age or of experience). One means of doing this is to invite group members to pair off and to verbalize, in those pairs, what they perceive to be the hidden agenda that they bring to the group. Such an activity can be rewarding in terms of the growth of the group but it is not recommended for the faint-hearted! Even if group members do not make explicit all of the hidden agenda that they bring to the group, the very act of taking part in the pairs activity will bring those agenda nearer to the surface.

All of these group processes commonly occur in groups of all sorts. They are, perhaps, more common in therapy and self-awareness groups but also crop up in learning groups. A useful way of exploring such processes is to use an exercise that involves the ground rules indicated below. A discussion held using these ground rules will often enhance the development of group processes and will also make them more noticeable to the group. After the discussion has been run for about an hour using the rules, they can be dropped and a discussion encouraged about what happened. The ground rules can also be adopted on a regular basis as a means of enhancing clear and assertive communication between group participants as follows.

Ground rules for a group discussion

- Say 'I', rather than 'you', 'we', or 'people' when discussing. Rather than say 'people in this group are getting a bit edgy', say 'I am getting a bit edgy'.
- Speak directly to other people rather than speaking about them. For example, rather than saying 'I think what John is saying is ...', say 'John, you seem to me to be saying that ...'.
- Avoid theorizing about what is happening in the group. Theorizing can often lead to a dry 'academic' discussion and can lead the group away from discussing how they are feeling as the group unfolds.
- Try to stay in the present tense: discuss what you are thinking and feeling **now**.

Genlin and Beebe offer another set of ground rules that may either be used as an alternative to the ones already cited, or they may be used alongside them. These ground rules have a broader application than the previous ones and are not value-free: they presuppose a particular view of groups. It is interesting to ponder on the degree to which you agree with their use in a health-care/interpersonal skills training context.

1. Everyone who is here belongs here just because he is here and for no other reason.
2. For each person what is true is determined by what is in him, what he directly feels and finds making sense in himself and the way he lives inside himself.
3. Our first purpose is to make contact with each other. Everything else we might want or need comes second.
4. We try to be as honest as possible and to express ourselves as we really are and really feel – just as much as we can.
5. We listen for the person inside – living and feeling.
6. We listen to everybody.
7. The group leader is responsible for two things only; he protects the belonging of every member and he protects their being heard if this is getting lost.
8. Realism: if we know things are a certain way, we do not pretend they are not that way.
9. What we say here is 'confidential': no one will repeat anything said here outside the group, unless it concerns only himself. This applies not just to obviously private things, but to everything. After all, if the individual concerned wants others to know something, he can always tell them himself.
10. Decisions made by the group need everyone taking part in some way.
11. New members become members because they walk in and remain. Whoever is here belongs (Gendlin and Beebe, 1968).

It is interesting to reflect on the degree to which you could use this set of ground rules in your own area of training. It is sometimes helpful to negotiate this second set of rules with the particular group and then such ground rules can serve as a group contract – to be adhered to by all group members for the life of the group.

Finally, Hobbs (1992) offers another set of guidelines for working with groups of the sort described in this book:

1. There will be no gossiping or discussion outside the training group about any personal material divulged by participants or about any person's performance during the sessions. All such information must be treated as confidential. This is to protect each individual as well as the whole group.
2. The training activities are not competitive. Each person must acknowledge that much learning arises from being open to examining 'what went wrong'.
3. All participants must acknowledge that they are each competent people/adults in their own right. Although personal involvement is without doubt a most valuable part of the group training experience, it is inappropriate to regard these training sessions as 'free personal therapy'. The trainers have a responsibility to offer effective training but each participant remains responsible for herself or himself (Hobbs, 1992).

It is interesting to note the similarities and differences between the suggested 'rules' for groups, between the list offered by Gendlin and Beebe in 1968 and that offered by Hobbs in 1992. While both lists seem to propose a liberal and democratic atmosphere and both indicate that what happens in groups should be deemed confidential to group members, Hobbs's list indicates a move away from the idea of learning groups as 'therapeutic'. It is arguable that Gendlin and Beebe's list more closely echoes the freethinking spirit of the 1960s in which it was conceived and that Hobbs's list adopts a rather more pragmatic 'training' approach. It is obvious, of course, that ideas about learning are always rooted in the cultural and historical situations in which they occur. The 'experiential' approach to running learning groups, as we have seen, grew most rapidly in the climate of the 1960s and 1970s. However, the principles of the approach have remained remarkably constant.

There is one area at least in which we may want to exercise caution and that is in the domain of the language we use when conducting experiential learning groups. In research that I have conducted into experiential learning (Burnard, 1992a), I have noted a tendency for some group facilitators to use the style of language that is most closely associated with learning groups of the 1960s. Examples of the use of such language include the clichés: 'may I share something with you?', 'I want to find out where you are coming from ...' and so on. It may be reasonable to argue that younger participants in experiential learning groups are likely to be either unfamiliar with such use of language or, possibly, embarrassed by it. It was notable, for instance, in my study of experiential group facilitators and students, that, while a number of the facilitators used language of this sort during interviews, students **never** used this sort of language during interviews. We would proably be wise, like Hobbs, to adapt our style of group facilitation to suit, at least in some ways, the times we find ourselves living in.

EMOTIONS AND GROUP WORK

The personal nature of experiential learning facilitation means that, sometimes, some participants will experience strong emotions. That is to say that on occasions, some may cry or get angry or even frightened. One argument is that some exercises 'restimulate' buried feelings. Another is that the exercises 'remind' some participants of earlier life events and cause them to experience strong feelings.

The facilitator who works, regularly, with experiential training methods needs to make a decision about whether or not to 'work' with these feelings. The term 'work' is used here to denote the idea of the facilitator helping the participant to release feelings or to resolve the issue that has arisen. There are various points of view about this issue and it is worth considering some of them.

First, is the view that the overt expression of emotion has no place in an educational encounter. The argument here is that education (or training) and 'therapy' – in its broadest sense – are two very different sorts of things. Therefore, education should be about learning knowledge and skills and no attempt should be made to engage with participants feelings. This argument involves the assumption that feelings can be separated out from our knowledge or skills.

Second, is the view that facilitating a group involves a tacit contract with that group. If the group members are expecting an educational experience and are 'contracted' with the facilitator to have such an experience, then the facilitator has no particular right to 'personalize' the group experience nor to involve the participants in expression of emotion. This is a variant of the position outlined in the previous paragraph.

A third view is that knowledge, skills and feelings are intimately bound up with one another and that any change in knowledge is likely to lead to a change in feelings. In this case, feelings cannot be ignored: they are an inevitable result of people learning things about themselves.

Yet another view is that education and therapy are part of the same activity. Therapy is a form of learning and experiential learning groups are part of a process of learning about yourself. As part of this equation, feelings are necessarily bound to surface and, in this case, the facilitator is duty bound to deal with them when they arise.

The facilitator, then, has to make a decision about what to do about the 'feelings issue'. This is not particularly straightforward. The facilitator may, for example, decide that, as a rule, she will not encourage participants to work with their feelings. While this rule may apply, she is likely to find that, on occasions, a participant **does** get upset. In this case, she needs to have a strategy worked out for dealing with this. We need, then, to consider what the options are, here. They appear to be as follows.

- The facilitator makes the decision that 'working with feelings' is an acceptable part of her role. In this case, she is advised to have some formal training in working with feelings. She is also advised to make it very clear to participants that this is the contract she has with them. Furthermore, she ought not to make the expression of feelings appear to be compulsory. Participants should freely choose whether or not they want to work in this way.
- The facilitator makes the decision that, as a rule, she will not work with feelings in the group. In this case, she avoids exercises and situations that are likely to raise the emotional climate of the group. However, she also remains open to the possibility of **some** emotion being expressed on some occasions. She may choose to have formal training in working with emotions or she may simply pick up the skills through attendance at various workshops as a participant. Either way, she is prepared for what she will do should someone burst into tears.
- The facilitator makes the decison that she definitely will not work with feelings. If a situation arises that looks as though it may result in the expression of overt emotion, she takes avoiding action. This may be through moving the discussion away from emotional issues, through calling a break in the proceedings or by inviting any apparently distressed participant to take a short break – perhaps in the company of another, supportive participant. This option is the 'classical' educational option.

Coping with feelings

What does the facilitator do when feelings **do** erupt in a learning group? Again, there are various options and, this time, they are organized in a heirarchical arrangement. In the following list of options, they range from 'working with emotions' to 'helping to calm the situation'. Which option or options the facilitator chooses will depend on the general decision that she has taken about working in groups – as outlined above. The following options assume that a participant has begun to cry during an exercise or discussion. Clearly, other emotions may be expressed, ranging from anger, through tears, to anxiety.

- **Option 1**. The facilitor allows the participant to have her full attention and the support of the group. The facilitator reminds the partipant that it is 'acceptable' to the group to express emotion. She also allows the further expression of emotion by taking no action that would stop it. She may also, gently, question the person about what is happening to him or her. She may also move her position in the group next to the participant and show, through eye contact and by holding the participant's hand, that she is 'with' the other person. She allows full expression of feeling and a period, afterwards, during which the participant can sit quietly and piece together the insights that often follow from overt expression of emotion. Generally, this style of facilitation takes some training and some experience if it is to be handled well. Arguably, too, the facilitator needs to have considered her own emotional status and be aware of her own areas of emotional frailty.

- **Option 2**. The facilitator moves next to the participant and sits beside him or her, perhaps holding his or her hand, but continues with the exercise or the discussion. In this way, the facilitator is acknowledging and allowing the expression of emotion but is not letting it impede the remaining work of the group. At all times, the facilitator stays with the participant until he or she is quieter and then returns to her original place in the group. This is a type of 'half-way' approach to working with emotions. While participants are 'allowed' to express emotions, those emotions are not fully 'worked through' in the group. The facilitator may offer to help the participant after the group has finished.

- **Option 3**. The facilitator sees that a participant is becoming upset by what is going on in the group and takes one or more of the following actions: (a) she calls for the group to take a short break and talks to the participant. It should be borne in mind that this type of intervention may cause the participant to release emotion during the break and the facilitator should be prepared for this; (b) she deftly and skilfully moves the subject of the discussion or exercise away from the current topic and allows the participant to 'recover'.

An example

If the facilitor does decide that the expression of feelings can be a norm in the group, she has a variety of strategies to choose from in working with those feelings. The following is an example of using a technique from Gestalt therapy to help a participant to explore a sudden search of emotion. In this example, the participants in the group have been discussing ways of helping children and young people when they have to stay in hospital. One of the group members suddenly begins to cry. The facilitator moves her position and sits next to the participant.

Facilitator: What's happening at the moment?
Participant: I feel very upset ... I keep crying.
Facilitator: What is the main feeling that goes with that?
Participant: I don't know. I feel odd.
Facilitator: Can you go back in time to when you felt like this before ...
Participant: Yes, I can remember a time ...
Facilitator: What I would like you to do is to describe, very carefully, and in detail, the situation that you were in, then ...
Participant: It was in the house at home, where I used to live ...

Facilitator: How old were you?

Participant: 16.

Facilitator: OK, describe the situation.

Participant: It was in the front room of the house. I can see it now. There is the old settee that we'd had for years ... the television set in the corner ... the chair my father always used to sit in .... My sister is in the room and we are arguing. I can't remember what about. I am upset with my sister because I feel that she always got her own way ... I felt my sister was treated differently by my parents and that she always got what she wanted. That used to upset me. [*The participant cries for a few minutes, then slowly stops and dries her eyes.*]

Facilitator: What are you feeling now?

Participant: (grins) Not so bad, now. I realize how dramatic I was then and how unreasonable it was to think that. Looking back, now, I realize that my parents didn't really treat my sister differently. But I've hung on to that for all this time! It makes more sense now. Thanks.

Facilitator: And how are you feeling now?

Participant: Fine, OK. I don't feel upset anymore. I just want to think things through a bit.

Facilitator: Where are you now?

Participant: Where am I? Oh, I see what you mean. I'm here, with the group, discussing working with children ... and I feel a lot easier!

The theory behind this intervention is this. The feelings in the present (tears) are linked to the topic under discussion (adolescence and childhood). The facilitator invites the participant to search through memories until he finds a situation in which he felt a similar emotion to the present one. This is then 're-lived' by the participant by describing, in some detail, the physical details of the situation. The participant, in re-living this situation, releases further emotion and re-evaluates his memory of it. He is then allowed to further think things through (a process that will go on after the group has finished) and then is gently 'brought back' to the present, by the facilitator.

This is a delicate area. Some participants in experiential groups are happy to express emotions fairly readily while others can be embarrassed by any show of feelings. The decision about whether or not the expression of emotion becomes a group norm is not one that is easily made and may, indeed, be made **for** the facilitator by a group member who is very suddenly distressed by something that happens during an activity. Perhaps, in the end, few hard and fast rules can be made here. It is vital, though, that any facilitator gives some thought to what she will do when emotion does arise in a group. She may not choose to follow the 'all emotional expressions are to be encouraged' but she is likely to experience the occasional situation in which her skills in handling feelings are put to the test.

In the end, decisions in this area are usually based on what the facilitator's beliefs are about the nature of emotion. Some, for instance, will believe that 'the expression of feelings is natural and helpful'. In this case, the facilitator will usually believe the complementary position that 'bottling up of feelings is unhelpful and potentially harmful'. Others, however, may take the view that the overt expression of emotion simply reinforces that action. In other words, when we cry or get angry, we simply learn how to become more effective at crying or getting angry. Yet other facilitors may take the view that sometimes the expression of emotion is helpful but that it is something that is mostly to be done in private and not as part of a learning group. Finally, the facilitator's personality comes into the equation. Not every facilitator will want or be able to handle other people's emotional release successfully and helpfully. For some, the expression of emotion, by others, can be difficult. It would be easy, here, to see some sort of direct link between the ease with which a person can handle other people's emotion and the degree to which they can handle their own. Such a link, however, has yet to be proved –although it is a popular belief among those who run groups in the humanistic field of group work.

SELF AND PEER EVALUATION

At the end of any learning encounter it is usual to undertake an appraisal in order to plan future learning sessions. The concept of self and peer evaluation has been alluded to in the discussion about both philosophical and practical aspects of experiential learning. Such an approach offers learners the chance to consider their own skills and learning and also to offer feedback on skills and learning to others. The approach is easily described and is best broken down into stages.

1. The learning group 'brainstorms' criteria for evaluation. These may or may not include such things as:

   - contribution to the group;
   - degree of self-awareness shown;
   - level of self-disclosure;
   - etc.

2. The list of criteria generated by the brainstorming session is prioritized and the first five criteria are selected as those suitable for use in the evaluation activity.
3. Each person in the group (including the facilitator) spends ten minutes on her own, considering her performance and levels of learning under the headings of the five criteria.
4. The group reforms and one person outlines their evaluation of themself, to the group.

5. That person then receives both negative and positive feedback from the group, under the five headings. This is the 'peer' element of the activity and is, like all other activities, voluntarily entered into. Some people may prefer not to receive peer feedback.

6. Once one person has undergone the self and peer review, the process moves onto the next person in the group and the cycle is repeated: first the individual offers the group her appraisal and evaluation, then the group offers feedback. As we have noted, the facilitator enters the evaluation process as an equal and does not necessarily have the first or the last word.

This process of self and peer evaluation takes time. Done properly, with a group of about ten people, it can occupy a whole afternoon. Done properly, however, it can be a valuable means of developing self-awareness and of forward planning for future learning activities. It may be used either as a form of formative evaluation or as a form of summative evaluation (Scriven, 1967). That is to say that it can be used in the middle of a course as a means of judging progress or it can be used at the end of a course as a method of deciding on the effectiveness and usefulness of the course.

FORMAL EVALUATION

Most educational and training organizations are now required to evaluate their courses more formally as part of an audit trail. The following is an example of a questionnaire that can be used at the end of an experiential workshop – in this case, on counselling. The questionnaire can easily be adapted to suit other sorts of workshops.

Course participants are given photocopies of the questionnaire on the last day of the workshop and asked to fill them in before they leave. They can, of course, be completed anonymously but it is important to make sure that every participant hands in a completed questionnaire. Participants simply tick the box after each question that most nearly matches their response to the item. After each item, there is space for more general comments. The example, below, illustrates a completed questionnaire.

Participants should be reminded to respond to every item and to tick only one box against each item. They should be instructed, too, that their responses will be treated in confidence and will help in the planning of future courses. This final point must, of course, be true – there is little point in asking for formal course feedback if the information obtained is not **used**. It is vital that the workshop leader collates the information gained from these questionnaires and uses it to guide future curriculum and workshop planning.

Brownstone College of Health and Science

Counselling Skills Workshop

Workshop Evaluation Form

We are committed to maintaining and strengthening the quality of the courses that we offer to participants. I would be grateful if you would take a few minutes to complete this form and to add any comments that you may have about how the Counselling workshop might be improved. Your comments will be discussed by the teaching staff and reported to the Board of Health Care Studies.

Andrew Brown
Workshop leader

---

1. I feel that the aims of the workshop have been achieved.

Strongly agree	Agree	Don't know	Disagree	Strongly disagree
1 ✓	2	3	4	5

Comments
I appreciated the fact that we were invited to identify some of our *own* aims for the workshop...
....
....
....

2. Varied teaching and learning methods have been used throughout the workshop.

Strongly agree	Agree	Don't know	Disagree	Strongly disagree
1	2 ✓	3	4	5

Comments
I enjoyed the exercises in pairs ....
....
....
....

3. Most students have taken an active part in the workshop.

Strongly agree	Agree	Don't know	Disagree	Strongly disagree
1 ✓	2	3	4	5

Comments

Two participants sometimes dominated the group ....
....
....
....

4. The quality of the teaching on this course was high.

Strongly agree	Agree	Don't know	Disagree	Strongly disagree
1	2	3 ✓	4	5

Comments

I have little experience – difficult to judge ....
....
....
....

5. The content of this workshop will help me in my work.

Strongly agree	Agree	Don't know	Disagree	Strongly disagree
1	2	3	4 ✓	5

Comments

I'm not sure that I will, automatically, be able to apply this ....
....
....
....

6. The lecture room/teaching accommodation was satisfactory.

Strongly agree		Agree	Don't know	Disagree	Strongly disagree
1	✓	2	3	4	5

Comments

....
....
....
....

7. Access to teaching accommodation was good and I was able to get to the sessions on time.

Strongly agree		Agree	Don't know	Disagree	Strongly disagree
1	✓	2	3	4	5

Comments

....
....
....
....

8. Generally, the workshop seems well organized.

Strongly agree		Agree	Don't know	Disagree	Strongly disagree
1	✓	2	3	4	5

Comments

I would have liked some more on breaking bad news but, generally, it was very interesting and useful...
....
....
....

9. Please identify below, any issues that you feel need to be addressed in order to improve the quality of the counselling workshop.

As a manager in the health service, I would like to have had more input on how to deal with difficult situations. The general counselling training, though, was excellent. I enjoyed the course and learned a lot from it. The exercises in pairs were particularly useful and I think I learned a lot about myself and about how bossy I can be, sometimes! ... There probably needs to be more *breaks* in the course

....

....

....

....

....

Thank you for your time,

Andrew Brown,

Workshop leader.

PROCESSING THE EVALUATION QUESTIONNAIRE

Having asked participants to complete the questionnaire, the next stage is to organize the data from them in ways that will make reading the 'results' possible. The first stage is to undertake frequency counts of the numbers of responses to each option following each of the items. This is easily achieved with a spreadsheet.

The first stage is to collate the findings from the questionnarie items into a table in a spreadsheet, as illustrated in Table 6.1.

The next stage is to ask the spreadsheet to run frequency counts for each column of the chart. When instucted this way, the spreadsheet program will compute how many '1's, '2's, '3's, '4's and '5's there were for each item and will sort these into what the spreadsheet calls 'bins'. From this process, it will be possible to see at a glance how the workshop participants scored their questionnaires – as in Table 6.2.

Table 6.1 Spreadsheet

	Quest 1	Quest 2	Quest 3	Quest 4	Quest 5	Quest 6	Quest 7	Quest 8
Participant 1	1	2	1	3	4	1	1	1
Participant 2	2	1	2	1	1	1	2	2
Participant 3	2	2	2	3	3	3	4	5
Participant 4	1	2	2	1	1	2	3	2
Participant 5	1	1	1	1	1	1	2	1
Participant 6	2	1	2	3	2	1	3	4
Participant 7	4	2	1	1	2	3	4	1
Participant 8	1	4	2	2	1	2	1	1
Participant 9	5	4	3	3	5	3	5	5
Participant 10	3	1	1	3	1	2	1	1

Table 6.2 Achievement of workshop's aims

Strongly agreed	4
Agreed	3
Didn't know	1
Disagreed	1
Strongly disagreed	1

If participants offer 'comments' under the questionnaire items, these can be brought together under a series of headings, as in the following example. For larger workshops and larger groups of participants, there are computer programs such as The Ethnograph, PinPoint and NUD✳IST that can be used for this purpose. For small groups, it is probably easiest to collate the comments by hand as not everyone will put comments under each of the items and many people will, perhaps, not offer comments at all.

Item 1: I feel that the aims of the workshop have been achieved

Comments

'I appreciated the fact that we were invited to identify some of our own aims for the workshop.'

'Too much time was spent in discussing the aims of the course. I felt we could have moved on a bit quicker.'

'The aims session was useful. It helped me to think about what we were doing.'

'The group was allowed to argue and debate too long. This seemed like a waste of time to me.'

'The main aims were clearly stated in the handout at the beginning of the workshop.'

OTHER EVALUATION METHODS

The types of methods of evaluating experiential learning activities described in this chapter are certainly not exhaustive of all possible methods. Packham, Roberts and Bawden (1989) identify a useful range of activities that they call 'validations' and which seem to span both elements of **assessment** and **evaluation**. Those validations were used to help in the assessment of students who work with various sorts of clients and could easily be adapted for use in health care settings. For them, validations may include:

1. feedback from the situation explored as to the client's reaction to the learner's approach and any outcomes of the project from their perspective;
2. reflections by the learner about the methodology used, techniques and skills developed, the process of learning itself, and what the project has meant to the learning has meant in terms of personal growth;
3. feedback from staff or other resource consultants on their use of particular concepts, methodologies, techniques and skills;
4. feedback from peers on their role as a group member, or other aspects the peer is qualified to comment on (Packham, Roberts and Bawden, 1989).

In a sense, the experiential learning facilitator is giving feedback all the time. She will be offering feedback after exercises, role plays and during and after discussions. Effective use of feedback is an essential part of the reinforcement process. If we want health professionals to develop a range of effective interpersonal skills then it is essential that the facilitator becomes something of an expert on giving feedback. French (1994) offers the following principles to improve the quality of feedback:

1. Feedback should be given in the form of description rather than an evaluation. Opinions, value judgements and guesses about the learner's motives are rarely helpful.
2. It should be constructive, not destructive. It should help the learner, not limit or restrict him.
3. It should be specific. Vague terminology or indirect reference to the behaviour in question tends to leave the learner in limbo. Feedback should be relevant and direct.
4. Feedback should be given about those aspects that are capable of change. If the person can really do nothing about the behaviour or attribute in question it will only cause conflict and emotional tension.
5. Feedback should be tactful and given in a climate of genuine concern and caring for the other person.

6. Reference to the behaviour should be made rather than reference to the person.
7. Feedback should be given at the person's request, not imposed upon him or her.
8. It should not normally always be one-sided. The teacher should allow the learner the opportunity to give feedback about the teacher's behaviour.
9. Feedback should be immediate and not delayed. It has reinforcing and motivating properties.
10. Feedback should be accurate and consistent. Over the long term, inconsistency from one person can be unsettling for the learner (French, 1994).

This chapter has taken a practical look at the processes involved in facilitating interpersonal skills groups. It has considered that process in stages, from the opening of the group to the final evaluation. It has also discussed some of the processes and dynamics that can occur in such groups and has offered two sets of ground rules for use in interpersonal skills work. The next stage in the process of learning about experiential learning in interpersonal skills development is to try it out! The next chapter describes how the exercises offered in the final chapter may be used.

7

Using experiential learning activities

This chapter offers concrete guidance on the use of the exercises for interpersonal skills development offered in the next chapter.

AIM OF THE ACTIVITY

In each of the exercise summaries in the next chapter, the intention of the activity is made clear. What can never be written for such exercises is a series of behavioural objectives. As we have noted throughout this book, experiential learning is necessarily idiosyncratic. It is not possible to predict the outcome of a particular exercise for any particular person. All that can be said is that there is a clear intention in setting out to offer the exercise as a learning activity.

NUMBER OF PARTICIPANTS RECOMMENDED

For most of the exercises, the minimum number of participants is probably four and there is no upper limit. However, with larger groups, the facilitator will have to consider bringing more structure to bear on the activities. He or she may, for example, want to produce printed handouts prior to undertaking the exercises, containing instructions about how to proceed. He or she may also want to identify some students as co-facilitators – people who can help in the arranging and setting up of the activities.

ENVIRONMENTAL CONSIDERATIONS

The usual suggestion, here, is that group members sit round in a circle. Such a circle is symbolic of unity and also ensures that the group facilitator is on an equal footing with the group and not physically (and symbolically) set apart from it. It is important, too, that the group does not sit around a table or in front of desks. In this way, there are no physical barriers between participants. The arrangement also allows for greater ease of movement if the exercise calls for the group's splitting into pairs or smaller groups.

EQUIPMENT REQUIRED

None of the exercises calls for difficult to obtain equipment. The most important feature of the exercises is the personal one: the meeting of people to enhance their skills. The equipment required for some exercises is a flip-chart pad, easel and flip chart marker pens. If these are not available, a blackboard or whiteboard is quite adequate. In some cases, no equipment at all is required.

ACQUIRING INTERPERSONAL SKILLS IN THE HEALTH PROFESSIONS: NUMBER 13

'New and good' exercise

Start an interpersonal skills group session off with a 'round' in which each person in turn reports something that has happened to them recently which is both 'new' and 'good'. This can be a useful and positive 'warmup' activity.

TIME REQUIRED

Taking time over these activities is very important. None of them should be rushed and plenty of time should be allowed for the discussional part of the activity.

THE ACTIVITY

This section, in each case, offers a clear, stage by stage account of how to run the exercise. Initially it is useful if these instructions are followed to the letter. Once the facilitator and the group have become familiar with the approach, various modifications can be made to suit the circumstances. Many of the most effective activities are those that the facilitator devises herself. On the other hand, as was noted above, it is important that none of the exercises is rushed.

EVALUATION PROCEDURE

Most of the following activities can best be evaluated by inviting the participants to take part in a pair of 'least and best' rounds. Two 'rounds' of the group
are instigated. In the first round, each person, in turn, states what he or she **least**
liked about the activity. In the second round, each person, in turn, states what he
or she **most** liked about the activity. A third round can be used in which each
person makes a statement about 'what I learned from this activity'. No discussion should take place **during** these rounds although the facilitator may or may
not choose to have a discussion **afterwards**. It is probably helpful if **everyone**
is encouraged to contribute in these rounds – including the facilitator.

WHEN TO USE THE EXERCISES

The activities described in the following chapter can be used, as they stand, in
workshops and other forms of interpersonal skills training. Combined with
icebreaker or other introductory exercises, they can form the basis of an entire
programme on aspects of interpersonal skills. They can also be combined with
more didactic sessions that consider theoretical and research aspects of interpersonal skills. Such theory inputs, it is suggested, should be kept short so as to
avoid the more traditional 'teacher centred' approach predominating. I have
found that a theory input can often be offered as a handout with headings, that
can serve as a discussional document. References to further reading can also be
supplied in this manner.

SEATING ARRANGEMENTS WITH SMALLER GROUPS

It is helpful if a fairly informal atmosphere can be generated in an interpersonal
skills training group. To this end, it is probably better that participants do not sit
behind desks or tables. Figures 7.1, 7.2 and 7.3 illustrate three possible chair
arrangements for a workshop. Figure 7.1, the 'three sides of a square' arrangement, is useful when numbers exceed 10–15. The arrangement allows all
students to see each other and encourages discussion among participants. It is,
perhaps, the most 'formal' of the arrangements and still leaves the group leader
very much 'in charge' of proceedings, at the front of the group.

The second arrangement, in two rows, gradually opening out (shown in
Figure 7.2), is useful for 'intermediate' sized groups and encourages discussion
between participants who are sitting next to each other and enables eye contact
to be maintained across the group. Again, it leaves the group leader at the front.
The third arrangement (Figure 7.3) is perhaps the most democratic. In the circle,
no one is perceived to be seated in any more 'important' seat than anyone else
and, symbolically, probably represents equality of membership. The group

leader can sit **anywhere** in the circle and may choose to sit in different places at different times.

One of the perennial problems with 'informal' seating arrangements is that once people move into pairs work, they often remain sitting in whatever part of the room they find themselves. It is a good idea to invite the group frequently to 'rearrange' itself into the original arrangement. Thus, if the circle is being used, it is helpful to suggest that gaps are closed and that the 'line' of the circle remains reasonably constant.

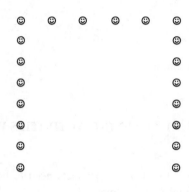

Figure 7.1 Seating arrangement 1

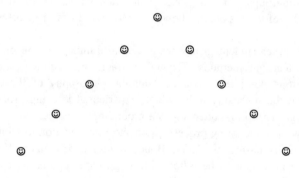

Figure 7.2 Seating arrangement 2

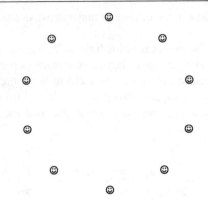

Figure 7.3 Seating arrangement 3

USING EXPERIENTIAL LEARNING ACTIVITIES WITH LARGER GROUPS

All but the most informal of learning projects need to be structured (Argyris, 1982). When experiential learning methods are used with larger groups, such structure becomes essential. In smaller groups, the facilitator normally takes care of the whole of the activity process. Thus, she will introduce an activity, make sure that the students are clear about their roles in that activity and then help them to make sense of it afterwards. With larger groups, this 'one-man band' approach may not be appropriate.

One obvious way of structuring the learning process is to divide up the group into small subgroups. Thus a group of 40 students can be divided into four groups of 10. Before this occurs, however, certain preparatory work needs to be done.

First, the larger student group needs a mini-training session on the use of experiential learning methods. Through a traditional lecture, followed by a discussion, it is possible to convey both the philosophy of the experiential approach and the mechanisms by which experiential learning groups operate. Thus the larger group of students gets a grounding in the personal and student-centred view of the learning process and a short introduction to facilitation and facilitation skills (Knowles, 1984; Boud, Keogh and Walker, 1985; Heron, 1990). These ideas can all be followed through with appropriate handouts and reading lists. It is suggested that this lecture and discussion are put into place early in an interpersonal skills or personal values course in order to prepare students for later experiential learning sessions. Also, it is important that extra rooms are booked early on. Dividing a larger group into subgroups is also going to mean that extra teaching space is required.

Once the initial introduction to the approach has been offered, a decision needs to be made about the degree to which the larger group will divide into smaller ones. One option is for the group to divide up and to stay in subgroups throughout the rest of the period of training. Another is that subgroups meet up at the end of any given training session and join a large plenary session. Yet another is that the student mix in the subgroups changes on a week-to-week basis, so that every student in the larger group gets to study with every other student. This type of decision can either be made by the tutor or lecturer, herself, or it can be discussed with the larger group and a more democratic approach used. Nor is there any reason why such a decision should be conclusive. It is quite possible to renegotiate the ground rules of this sort of activity as the tutor or lecturer gets a clearer idea of how the process is unfolding. Different divisions and groupings may also suit different cohorts of students.

RUNNING THE SMALLER GROUPS

When the larger group meets for their first training session, each subgroup will need a student-facilitator. If this topic has been discussed in some detail at the initial lecture and discussion, the election of such a student-facilitator should cause few problems. If it seems likely that there will be a problem, the tutor or lecturer might elect to choose such facilitators herself. The role of the student-facilitator will include the following elements:

- describing the experiential learning activity to the group and giving them appropriate handouts containing explicit instructions;
- ensuring the smooth running of the activity;
- enabling the discussion of the activity after it has occurred;
- feeding back to the larger plenary group where this is appropriate.

The tutor or lecturer's task in organizing the smaller groups will include, at least, the following elements:

- the preparation of clear handouts that give detailed but straightforward instructions about the task in hand;
- ensuring that the subgroups find their rooms and are clear about the subgroups they are to join;
- facilitating the larger plenary session when this is appropriate;
- ensuring that the student-facilitators are adequately supervised and that their own learning needs are met;
- making sure that learning is appropriately assessed and evaluated. It is vital that transfer of learning takes place, from the experiential learning group to the clinical setting. Self and peer review and the use of diaries as monitors of the transfer of learning have both been described in the literature (Kilty, 1978; Burnard, 1987; Boud, Keogh and Walker, 1985).

The tutor or lecturer may also choose from three other options. She may join one of the subgroups as a participant (or as a stand in for an absent student-facilitator). She may spend some time with each of the groups and move between them during the course of a session. She may, on the other hand, leave the groups to work on their own. Of all of these options, the second is perhaps the least appropriate. Although the idea of 'overseeing' groups of students is often advocated during teacher preparation, in experiential learning groups it seems more likely to be an intrusion and an interruption than a help. Perhaps the best option is the first one. If the tutor or lecturer can join in a sub-group as a participant, she is not only role-modelling effective group membership but she is also further perpetuating the adult-learning principles of experiential learning by being a 'co-traveller' in the learning process (Jarvis, 1987). On the other hand, such an idea of equality can be taken too far. While teachers and students can learn together, it is usually clear from their ages, professional experience and training, that they are also not equal in many ways. This, too, should be recognized and the tutor or lecturer should be sensitive about the degree to which she can be recognized as an 'equal' by the learning group.

STUDENT-FACILITATORS

The task of being a student-facilitator is not a particularly easy one. The student is being asked to be both a peer and a learning facilitator. It should be pointed out, though, that she is not being asked to be a teacher. The role should not necessitate any formal teaching input. Instead, it involves the organization and processing of a particular experiential learning activity. The aim is not to turn students into teachers but to enable students to work more effectively as facilitators of learning. Also, by role-modelling such facilitation, it seems likely that those student-facilitators are also conveying to their peers a certain set of attitudes both towards learning and towards people in general. Also, as Infante (1986) pointed out, health care teachers, themselves, are constantly role-modelling the teaching and facilitation role. Teachers who adopt the approaches outlined in this section should frequently reflect on the style of facilitation that they are modelling.

It seems reasonable that the role should not be thrust upon any given student. Instead, students should be free to elect to take up the role. In the early stages of this approach, it is likely that only the more extrovert members of the group will take up the challenge. As the subgroups develop, however, the task is likely to be seen as more 'manageable' by other, less assertive members. It also seems unlikely that every student will be able to (or want to) act in this capacity during the life of one course of training and education.

It is essential, too, that the student-facilitators are also able to identify the learning that they develop from the role. It is helpful if all of the student-facilitators meet for a plenary session of their own, with the tutor or lecturer. In such a session, the students can be debriefed and can talk through their experiences of both facilitating the small groups and of learning through running a group. Quite often, the timing element of the task presents problems. The experiential learning activity often overruns in the early stages of the subgroup formation and the student-facilitator is not left enough time to process that activity. At this point, the tutor or lecturer can offer assistance as to how time may be used more effectively. Also, the tutor should make sure, beforehand, that the timings on her handout are realistic. It is one thing to plan out an experiential learning activity but another to ensure that it runs to time.

NON-PEER FACILITATORS

Another approach to working with larger student groups is to invite students who are **not** peers, to run the smaller groups. In this approach, senior students are invited to work as facilitators in these groups and thus enhance their own group and facilitation skills. The same sort of preparation of student-facilitators is required but senior students may be better prepared to adopt the role by virtue of their own previous training in group facilitation. This assumes, of course, that group facilitation is on the curriculum in the first place. If it is not, the preparation of the facilitators will almost exactly mimic that of peer facilitators.

There are advantages and disadvantages of using students from other years or other groups. Outside facilitators can sometimes be more objective and more able to run the group smoothly and effectively. They may also bring more experience to the task than peer facilitators might. On the other hand, in running other students' groups, they are clearly going to have to forfeit doing something else. Careful organization may be necessary to ensure that non-peer facilitators do not feel that they are being 'used'. The advantages and value of being encouraged to run groups in this way must be made apparent to the students concerned.

OTHER ISSUES

The two approaches to learning, described here, offer ways of furthering the idea of adult learning in health care education. They also ask that the tutor or lecturer be prepared to give up part of her organizing and controlling role. Asking students to work in this way means that learning outcomes are likely to be less predictable. Just as it is unreasonable to set behavioural objectives for more 'traditional' experiential learning activities, so is it also less than useful to do so in these situations. However, some tutors or lecturers may want to encourage students to write their own, expressive, objectives before they start working in the small groups or before they take on the role of student-facilitator.

Linked to all this is the need to be able to evaluate learning effectively. Here, it seems likely that self and peer evaluation will be appropriate, as will be some format for assessing the effectiveness of the supervision offered by the tutor or lecturer to the student-facilitators (Bodley, 1992). In the longer term, both course and lecturer evaluation will be necessary (MacDonald, 1992). As we have noted, too, it is of considerable importance that any learning that takes place in these groups is linked to the 'real world' of the students' everyday clinical experience. The point is not merely to discuss a range of issues, nor to practise a range of skills but to identify how and why such issues and skills related to nursing.

Once this form of educational activity has become established in a given college of health care, it may be felt advisable to introduce short training courses within the mainstream course, to enable all students to develop the skills of facilitation more formally. Such skills will not be wasted. Facilitation skills are being more widely advocated as part of the range of skills that any health care professional can use in clinical and community settings (Robinson and Vaughan, 1992). Also, the notion of peer teaching is being discussed, increasingly, in the nursing education literature as an appropriate way of helping students to learn (Costello, 1989; Clarke and Feltham, 1990). Students also need to be encouraged to discuss the relative differences between the concepts of teaching (the passing on of information) and facilitation (helping and encouraging others to learn through reflection).

Clearly, too, there are other educational issues at stake in using methods such as these. It is important, for example, that students who are trained as facilitators are allowed to discuss, in some detail, the principles of experiential learning. They need time to be allowed to 'own' these ideas and to be motivated to help each other to learn. In a study of nearly 500 students' and tutors' perceptions of experiential learning methods, Burnard (1991) found that many students (and a number of nurse teachers) found some experiential learning methods embarrassing to use. It is important that teachers who are helping to train student-facilitators allow those students enough time to air their anxieties and doubts about the approaches.

Finally, it is also possible to run experiential learning activities with large groups who stay together. While the idea of working in smaller groups is preferable, there seems to be no reason why an experienced tutor or lecturer could not facilitate the group as a whole. However, most writers on the topic of experiential learning facilitation stress the importance of the small group format as a means of ensuring student participation and the exchange of ideas and feelings (see, for example, Heron, 1973; Kilty, 1983). If the larger group format is used, then much thought has to go into the organization of activities. Very clear structure is likely to be required if the group is to stay together.

This section has described two approaches to helping students to learn from experience in large groups. Both involve the use of other students as facilitators. Both uphold the principles of adult learning which acknowledge an equality in the roles of facilitators and students. Both need careful planning but such planning can help to ensure that interpersonal skills do not get 'taught' only through lectures and discussion. The methods encourage full participation and enable reflection on a wide range of communication and interpersonal skills appropriate to any nursing course. Nor are the methods limited to experiential learning. They could easily be adapted for more 'formal' elements of a course and used as method of structuring small group teaching and learning in both post and preregistration courses.

RECORDING INTERPERSONAL SKILLS ACTIVITIES

If you run interpersonal skills training sessions on a regular basis, it makes sense to keep records of the activities that you use. These can be useful for planing sessions in the future, for recording student responses to various activities and for modifying activities for use in different situations and contexts. Such records can either be kept in a notebook or are ideally suited for keeping in a **freeform database** on a personal computer. A freeform database differs from a **flatfile** or **relational** database in that you can enter as much or as little information in each 'form' or record as you need. Unlike the flatfile or relational database, you do not have to specify, in advance, the format or structure of your records.

Two, typical, examples of freeform database programs for the personal computer are **Idealist** (Blackwell, 1993) and **askSam**. Both programs allow you to enter information as plain text, either in a structured or semi-structured format or simply as typed-in text. You are then free to look up whatever aspects of your records you require. It is usually a good idea to have at least minimal structure for your records and a typical layout for **Idealist** may be as illustrated in Figure 7.4.

The real value of the **freeform database** approach to storing information about activities is that new information, of any amount, can be added to each record. Over a period of time, for example, the 'notes' section and the 'contexts' section may grow considerably. A flatform or relational database program would restrict you to a certain number of characters in each entry (usually 256 characters per field). Programs such as **Idealist** and **askSam** have no such restrictions. Indeed, **askSam** has almost no limit to the amount of text that can be included in each record. The layout in **askSam** is different to that of **Idealist** and each record in it looks more like a page in a wordprocessor. An **askSam** record (using the same information as contained in the **Idealist** program) would look like this. What separates the 'fields' in an **askSam** record is the square bracket ([ ) as illustrated in Figure 7.5.

Both programs allow you to print out any parts of your records that you need and to quickly search for various sorts of activities. You might, for example, search for all of the activity records that you have on listening or all of the

Name of the activity	Simple listening in pairs
Aim of the activity	To encourage participants to explore listening to others
Number of participants required	Any even number between 6 and 20
Environmental considerations	Useful to have large room or rooms in which participants can spread out. Chairs of equal height. Don't forget to encourage participants to choose different people when they do this activity more than once.
The process	Participants pair off. Each is nominated 'A' and 'B'. A listens for 5 minutes while 'B' talks. Afterwards, pairs swap roles and continue for further 5 minutes. Plenary session.
Notes	Use 'neutral' topics with 'new groups'. Remember to remind participants to notice when they 'dry up' and to observe what they do about it! Remind, if necessary, to keep to the rules of the exercise and not to turn it into a conversation. Allow plenty of time for plenary.
Participant reactions	Mostly positive. One student in a physiotherapy course said she 'couldn't see the point' and refused to take part in further exercises. Generally goes down well at the beginning of counselling courses. Some groups prefer you to suggest topics.
Dates used	12.4.95; 14.5.95; 6.8.95; 2.9.95.
Contexts	1st year nursing students workshop. Physiotherapy 'training the trainers' course. Back to nursing course. Various weekend workshops, multidisciplinary.

Figure 7.4 Example layout of an 'activities' record in **Idealist**

activities that you used on a certain date at a certain workshop. In this way, you can consult your activities database when planning a workshop or training session and print out the required activities. You can also store participant hand-outs in the database and print these out too. Both programs have their strengths and deficits. **Idealist** has a smarter interface and is more obviously easy to use once it is set up. Setting up, though, is not particularly intuitive and most users have to spend a little time reading the manual. **askSam** is not quite so smart to look at but is much more powerful than Idealist both in terms of the amount of data that it can hold and in its **searching** facilities. **askSam** is probably easier to set up, initially. Both programs, though, are simple to use once you have learned a little about them.

I have found it useful to use both of them. I keep my bibliographical references and names and address lists in Idealist and use askSam for keeping details

Name of the activity	[Simple listening in pairs
Aim of the activity	[To encourage participants to explore listening to others
Number of participants required	[Any even number between 6 and 20
Environmental considerations	[Useful to have large room or rooms in which participants can spread out. Chairs of equal height. Don't forget to encourage participants to choose different people when they do this activity more than once.
The process	[Participants pair off. Each is nominated 'A' and 'B'. 'A' listens for 5 minutes while 'B' talks. Afterwards, pairs swap roles and continue for further 5 minutes. Plenary session.
Notes	[Use 'neutral' topics with 'new groups'. Remember to remind participants to notice when they 'dry up' and to observe what they do about it! Remind, if necessary, to keep to the rules of the exercise and not to turn it into a conversation. Allow plenty of time for plenary.
Participant reactions	[Mostly positive. One student in a physiotherapy course said she 'couldn't see the point' and refused to take part in further exercises. Generally goes down well at the beginning of counselling courses. Some groups prefer you to suggest topics.
Dates used	[12.4.95; 14.5.95; 6.8.95; 2.9.95.
Contexts	[1st year nursing students workshop. Physiotherapy 'training the trainers' course. Back to nursing course. Various weekend workshops, multidisciplinary.

Figure 7.5 Example layout of an 'activities' record in **askSam**

and notes about interpersonal skills training activities as outlined in this chapter. I also find **askSam** an invaluable program for handling textual data in qualitative research and used it in the analysis of interview data in the study on counselling discussed in Chapter 3.

The programs discussed in this section run on personal computers (IBMs or IBM compatibles) with a 386 or faster processor and a minimum of 4Mb of RAM. They both run under **Microsoft Windows** operating system. Both require a hard disk for optimal performance and – as with other **Windows** programs – are designed for use with a mouse.

QUESTIONS: PITFALLS AND PROBLEMS

Activities in groups are always different to the way they are described in books. No two groups are the same and what suits one group of people may not suit another. There are bound to be uncertainties about procedure and about group activity on the part of both facilitator and group members. It is often this 'uncertainty' element that makes groups interesting and a powerful source of learning. In the closing section of this chapter, various questions are posed about experiential learning activities and group procedure. They are ones frequently asked in training groups for facilitators and a variety of possible solutions is offered for each one.

What happens if the learners don't want to join in?

It is important that all of these activities is entered into voluntarily. No one should be forced to undertake an activity against their will. If a relaxed and informal atmosphere is maintained, most people will find the activities useful and interesting.

What happens if no one says anything during the discussional period?

This is where the use of a flip-chart pad or blackboard can help. If the facilitator is clearly prepared to make notes on what happens, then people's contributions to a discussion are seen to be valued. On the other hand, sometimes the use of such jotting down can serve to break up the discussion and in some cases, this approach should be abandoned in favour of free discussion. The keyword, here, is flexibility. It is important that the facilitator listens to what the group wants and needs and modifies the programme and the activities to suit that group.

What if one person talks too much in a discussion?

The facilitator has a number of options here:

1. She can allow the person to carry on overtalking and allow the group to deal with the issue.
2. She can 'shut out' the person, gently by holding up her hand and by drawing in other members of the group.
3. She can raise the issue of contributions made by group members, with the group and allow the issue of the dominant person to emerge,
4. She can directly confront the person and gently indicate that he is overtalking.

What if someone gets emotional during an exercise?

Sometimes some experiential learning activities can generate emotion. Again, the facilitator has a number of options available to her.

1. She can make a contract with the group, at the beginning of the session, to the effect that the expression of emotion is 'allowed' or even that it may be encouraged. This option is best used by someone who has had training in coping with emotional release. Courses on coping with cathartic release are offered by a growing number of colleges and extra-mural departments of universities.
2. She can note the developing emotional involvement and can switch the topic of conversation to a lighter note, so that emotional release is avoided.
3. She can acknowledge both to the individual and to the group, that emotions are rising and can ask the individual and/or the group what they wish to happen.

ACQUIRING INTERPERSONAL SKILLS IN THE HEALTH PROFESSIONS: NUMBER 14

Guidelines for effective experiential facilitation

1. Allow plenty of time.
2. Explain the activity clearly.
3. Make sure that the 'processing' period, after the activity is twice as long as the period taken up by the activity, itself.
4. Listen to participants and do not force a particular point of view on to them.
5. Make sure that all participation is voluntary.
6. Modify activities to suit this group at this time.

What if the facilitator feels that things are getting out of control?

This issue is usually linked to the previous one and relates to emotional expression by one or members of the group. A simple method of coping with this is to 'lighten' the atmosphere with a change of activity or a change of pace. Alternatively, the facilitator can suggest that the group takes a short break and that everybody be allowed a 'cooling-off' period.

What happens if the group falls silent?

This issue is considered in one of the exercises in group facilitation. Invariably there will be periods of silence in a group workshop. Sometimes, the silence 'feels' comfortable and is a necessary lull in the procedings. At other times, the silence feels hostile and it is helpful if the facilitator can confront the silence and invite the group to offer thoughts about why the silence has occurred or perhaps to invite questions about any 'hidden agendas' that may be at work in the group. Also, the silence may indicate a natural pause in the proceedings, signalling time for a change of activity or a break. Finally, a silence can indicate a loss of direction, by the facilitator, by the group, of both. Sometimes it can be helpful to disclose that you are lost in such circumstances: self-disclosure at times such as these can indicate that like all other members of the group, you are human and need help at times!

What happens if someone walks out of the group?

Again, there can be many reasons for a person leaving the group unannounced: tension, embarrassment, heightened emotion, boredom, hostility, a forgotten appointment and so forth. It is helpful if a decision is made prior to starting a learning group about whether or not people should be free to leave when they choose. If the agreement is that people can leave, then nothing, normally, need be done if someone walks out. On the other hand, if the agreement is that no one leaves without indicating their intention to do so, it may be helpful to send someone to talk to the person who absences themselves without warning. It is rarely helpful for the facilitator to leave the group to speak to the person who walks out. On the other hand, there will always be exceptions to these guidelines: unusual situations call for unusual interventions!

Can the activities be used in groups smaller in number than six?

Generally, the activities described here require a reasonably sized group (between 6 and 24) to enable the experiential learning cycle to be fully worked through. On the other hand, a number of the activities, including those concerned with counselling, assertiveness and social skills, can be carried out in pairs. If they are carried out between two people, it is important to stick to the structure of the activity and allow plenty of time for discussion of the acitivity after it has finished.

Does interpersonal skills training have to be all experiential learning?

No, ring the changes. The occasional formal lecture to fill in background information or to deepen group participants' thinking about a certain aspect of interpersonal relations can be very useful. On the other hand, lecturing can be seductive! It can be tempting and easy to slip back into the traditional 'information-giving' mode of the teacher or lecturer. Sometimes it is far more difficult to remain a facilitator than it is to return to a more familiar approach to teaching and learning. The pull is often in two directions: (1) the group seems to be asking for information and for a lecture; and (2) it seems appropriate to 'give in' and hand out information. It is often helpful to discuss this occurrence with the group as it happens, rather than just slip back into information-giving.

Do I have be trained in using experiential learning methods?

Experience in a variety of group situations is an advantage when using experiential learning activities. Experience of this sort can be gained in a number of ways. First, the would-be facilitator can take part in as many different types of group as possible, as a member. This will allow her to study other people's facilitation style and to observe group dynamics and how they are dealt with. Second, a number of colleges and extra-mural departments of universities offer short workshops on facilitating groups. These tend to run either for one or two days or for a full week. Thirdly, more formal training can be undertaken via enrolment of a part- or full-time course in group work. Again, such courses are offered by various colleges and universities and also by certain organizations specializing in particular sorts of group therapy, e.g. gestalt, psychodynamic or analytical therapies. Such courses are usually advertised in health service journals and in journals about groups and about psychotherapy. I have found a balance between formal training, attending occasional workshops and informally finding out as I go along a useful way to proceed. Again, it is a question of lifelong and experiential learning. No one ever stops learning about groups and group facilitation.

The next chapter of this book offers a range of exercises for interpersonal skills training. The exercises have all been used by the author in a variety of contexts and always with health care professionals. They are representative of a wide range of activities for encouraging the development of interpersonal skills, using the experiential learning approach, but are clearly not exhaustive of all possible types of exercises that can be used. More can be found in the items contained in the further reading list at the end of the book. The experiential way of working has been interesting, rewarding and always surprising: the exercises here work for me and I hope they will work for you too.

8 | Experiential learning activities for health professionals

ACTIVITY NUMBER 1

Aim of the activity

To identify basic interpersonal skills.

The activity

The larger group breaks into smaller subgroups of between six and ten members. A leader for each subgroup is elected and each subgroup addresses the following questions:

- What are the interpersonal skills that we use most frequently in our everyday work?
- How did we learn them?

Group participants' comments are jotted onto flip-chart sheets and, after 15 to 20 minutes, the larger group reconvenes. The facilitator pins up the flip-chart sheets and a plenary discussion is held with the whole group.

ACTIVITY NUMBER 2

Aim of the activity

To identify what gets in the way of being interpersonally effective.

The activity

The group breaks into pairs, who distribute themselves around the room. Each pair nominates one person as A and the other person as B. A then asks B, 'What gets in the way of your being as interpersonally effective as you would like to be?' and listens to the answer. If necessary, A repeats the question but does not join in any discussion about it. After five minutes, the pairs change round and B asks A the same question and listens to the answer.

After a further five minutes, the larger group reconvenes and a plenary discussion is held.

ACTIVITY NUMBER 3

Aim of the activity

To explore participants' experiences of effective communication.

The activity

This activity is based loosely on an activity described by Moustakas in his book about phenomenological research methods (1994). The group members are invited to sit, silently, for three minutes and to recall **a person whom each identifies as being an 'effective communicator'**. This person might be a personal friend, a teacher, a manager or any other person that the group member knows. As group members think about that person, they are encouraged to consider every aspect of the person: thus they might consider:

- what the person looks like,
- how he or she dresses,
- how he or she talks,
- his or her mannerisms,
- his or her 'negative' qualities, and so on.

After the silent four minutes, group participants are asked to jot down notes under the following headings:

- What the person was **like**
- What they did
- The **context of the relationship** (student/teacher, friend/friend etc.)
- What made them a good communicator
- The person's effect on **me**.

After a further period of ten minutes, the group divides up into small subgroups of no more than five people. Each subgroup shares the information they have gathered as individuals and develops a profile of an 'excellent communicator'. After a period of half an hour in the subgroups, the larger group reconvenes and the facilitator draws up a 'larger' profile of the 'excellent communicator'.

ACTIVITY NUMBER 4

Aim of the activity

To identify what participants need to do to improve their interpersonal skills.

The activity

The group divides into pairs. Each pair nominates one of them as A and the other as B. A then asks of B: 'what do you need to do to improve your interpersonal skills?' and listens to the answer without interruption. The question can be repeated, if necessary. After five minutes, the pair switch round and B asks the question of A. After a further five minutes, the larger group reconvenes and a plenary session is held to discuss responses to the question.

ACTIVITY NUMBER 5

Aim of the activity

To identify work situations in which good interpersonal skills are essential.

The activity

The group either works on this exercise as a whole or breaks into smaller subgroups. The aim is to identify, through 'brainstorming', which of the interpersonal skills available to health professionals are vital in the particular profession in which participants practise. The points are brainstormed onto large flip-chart sheets and after 15 minutes, a plenary discussion is evoked by the facilitator.

ACTIVITY NUMBER 6

Aim of the activity

To practise introductions.

The activity

The group pairs off. Each person in each of the pairs 'experiments' with introducing him or herself to his or her partner. He or she may try **any** sort of introduction, ranging from the abrupt and rude to the obsequious. The aim is to identify the key skills involved in successful introduction. After one person in each pair has tried a range of introductions, the pairs switch round and the other person introduces him or herself to his or her partner. After 15–20 minutes, the group reconvenes for a plenary session.

ACTIVITY NUMBER 7

Aim of the activity

To practise answering the phone.

The activity

The group divides up into pairs. Each pair sits back to back and practises 'answering the phone', using a range of approaches. In each case, one of the pair is the 'caller' and the other the 'answerer'. The aim is to identify appropriate and skilled methods of answering a call. Each member of each pair should practise a range of approaches to phone answering. After 10–15 minutes, the larger group reconvenes and a discussion is facilitated by the group leader.

ACTIVITY NUMBER 8

Aim of the activity

To practise starting an interview.

The activity

The group divides into pairs. One of each pair is 'interviewer' and the other is 'interviewee'. The interviewer, in his or her own time, tries out a range of 'openings' for an interview. These openings should be practised slowly and repeated as necessary so that 'fine tuning' can take place. After 15 minutes, the pairs swap roles and after a further 15 minutes, the pairs reconvene into a larger group to discuss the activity.

ACTIVITY NUMBER 9

Aim of the activity

To explore **not** listening to another person.

The activity

The group breaks up into pairs and the pairs move to various parts of the room so that they are not immediately overheard by other pairs. In each pair, one person is nominated A and the other B. A then talks to B for five minutes about any subject, while B **does not listen** to them! After five minutes, roles are reversed and A sits while B talks and A does not listen.

After a second five minutes, the group reconvenes and group members discuss what it was like not to be listened to. These comments may be jotted down onto a flip-chart sheet, white or blackboard, by the facilitator.

ACTIVITY NUMBER 10

Aim of the activity

To explore listening to another person.

THE ACTIVITY

The group breaks up into pairs and the pairs move to various parts of the room so that they are not immediately overheard by other pairs. In each pair, one person is nominated A and the other B. A then talks to B for five minutes about any subject, while B **listens** to them. After five minutes, roles are reversed and A sits while B talks and A listens. It is important that the pairs are told that this activity is not a conversation and that the partner's role is one of listening only.

After a second five minutes, the group reconvenes and group members discuss what it was like to be listened to. These comments may be jotted down onto a flip-chart sheet, white or blackboard, by the facilitator.

ACTIVITY NUMBER 11

Aim of the activity

To practise 'noticing'.

The activity

The concept of 'noticing', as described in the text of this book, is described to group members. The group breaks up into pairs and the pairs move to various parts of the room so that they are not immediately overheard by other pairs. In each pair, one person is nominated A and the other B. A then talks to B for five minutes about any subject, while B listens to them and practises 'noticing', as the other person talks. B should be instructed to notice everything that is going on, both inside herself and in the environment immediately in front of her. After five minutes, roles are reversed and A sits whilst B talks and A listens and notices.

After a second five minutes, the group reconvenes and group members discuss what it was like to be listened to. These comments may be jotted down onto a flip-chart sheet, white or blackboard, by the facilitator.

ACTIVITY NUMBER 12

Aim of the activity

To practise asking questions of another person.

The activity

The group breaks up into pairs and the pairs move to various parts of the room so that they are not immediately overheard by other pairs. In each pair, one person is nominated A and the other B. A then asks open and closed questions of B about any subject, while B listens to those questions, but does not allow the exercise to become a conversation. After five minutes, roles are reversed and B asks open and closed questions of A.

After a second five minutes, the group reconvenes and group members discuss what happened during the exercise. These comments may be jotted down onto a flip-chart sheet, white or blackboard, by the facilitator.

ACTIVITY NUMBER 13

Aim of the activity

To practise the use of 'reflection'.

The activity

The group breaks up into pairs and the pairs move to various parts of the room so that they are not immediately overheard by other pairs. In each pair, one person is nominated A and the other B. A then talks to B for ten minutes about any subject, while B practises the use of 'reflection'. After ten minutes, roles are reversed.

After a second ten minutes, the group reconvenes and group members discuss what happened during the activity. These comments may be jotted down onto a flip-chart sheet, white or blackboard, by the facilitator.

ACTIVITY NUMBER 14

Aim of the activity

To practise a combination of facilitative interventions.

The activity

The group breaks up into pairs and the pairs move to various parts of the room so that they are not immediately overheard by other pairs. In each pair, one person is nominated A and the other B. A then initiates a conversation with B and uses **only** facilitative interventions (open questions, closed questions, reflections or empathy-building statements), during that conversation. After ten minutes, roles are reversed and B initiates a conversation with A, using only facilitative interventions during that conversation.

After a second ten minutes, the group reconvenes and group members discuss what happened during the activity. These comments may be jotted down onto a flip-chart sheet, white or blackboard, by the facilitator.

ACTIVITY NUMBER 15

Aim of the activity

To explore counselling badly.

The activity

The group breaks up into pairs and the pairs move to various parts of the room so that they are not immediately overheard by other pairs. In each pair, one person is nominated A and the other B. A spends ten minutes using a range of counselling skills **as badly as possible**! After that ten minutes, roles are reversed and B counsels A, using counselling skills as badly as possible! The aim in each case should be to demonstrate how counselling should not be prac-tised.

After a second ten minutes, the group reconvenes and group members discuss what happened during the activity. These comments may be jotted down onto a flip-chart sheet, white or blackboard, by the facilitator.

ACTIVITY NUMBER 16

Aim of the activity

To identify personal counselling skills.

The activity

The group breaks up into pairs and the pairs move to various parts of the room so that they are not immediately overheard by other pairs. In each pair, one person is nominated A and the other B. Each pair then spends ten minutes identifying what they consider are their strengths and weaknesses as counsellors. Each person, in each pair, invites the other person to assess her strengths and weaknesses as well as undertaking a personal assessment.

After ten minutes, the group reconvenes and group members discuss what happened during the activity. These comments may be jotted down onto a flip-chart sheet, white or blackboard, by the facilitator. The items identified during this activity may then be used as the basis of a counselling skills workshop.

ACTIVITY NUMBER 17

Aim of the activity

To practise introductions and closure in a counselling session.

The activity

The group breaks up into pairs and the pairs move to various parts of the room so that they are not immediately overheard by other pairs. In each pair, one person is nominated A and the other B. A then practises opening a counselling session with B. Participants should be encouraged to explore a wide range of expressions, phrases and approaches in order to discover what suits them and what does not. A then practises closing the counselling session, again spending time practising a wide range of possibilities. After ten minutes, A and B swap roles and B practises openings and closings with A.

After ten minutes, the group reconvenes and group members discuss what happened during the activity. These comments may be jotted down onto a flip-chart sheet, white or blackboard, by the facilitator.

ACTIVITY NUMBER 18

Aim of the activity

Exploring silence.

The activity

The group breaks up into pairs and the pairs move to various parts of the room so that they are not immediately overheard by other pairs. In each pair, one person is nominated A and the other B. Each pair then spends ten minutes sitting facing each other in total silence. Each person is encouraged to reflect on how they feel about the silence and to note what physical and behavioural mani-festations the silence brings about.

After ten minutes, the group reconvenes and group members discuss what happened during the activity. These comments may be jotted down onto a flip-chart sheet, white or blackboard, by the facilitator.

ACTIVITY NUMBER 19

Aim of the activity

To explore aspects of assertiveness.

The activity

The group breaks up into pairs and the pairs move to various parts of the room so that they are not immediately overheard by other pairs. In each pair, one person is nominated A and the other B. Then A sits opposite B and says 'yes' to them. B replies 'no'. The pairs are encouraged to explore the use of these two words with various tones and volumes of voice. The activity must not involve conversation, but only the words 'yes' and 'no'. After five minutes, roles are reversed and A says 'no' to B's 'yes'.

After a second five minutes, the group reconvenes and group members discuss what happened during the activity. These comments may be jotted down onto a flip-chart sheet, white or blackboard, by the facilitator. The group also explores how individual members cope with saying 'no' to other people.

ACTIVITY NUMBER 20

Aim of the activity

To explore aspects of assertiveness.

The activity

The group breaks up into pairs and the pairs move to various parts of the room so that they are not immediately overheard by other pairs. In each pair, one person is nominated A and the other B. Then A sits opposite B and says 'I want to' to them. B replies 'you can't'. The pairs are encouraged to explore the use of these two phrases with various tones and volumes of voice. The activity must not involve conversation, but only the two phrases. After five minutes, roles are reversed and A says 'you can't' to B's 'I want to'.

After a second five minutes, the group reconvenes and group members discuss what happened during the activity. These comments may be jotted down onto a flip-chart sheet, white or blackboard, by the facilitator.

ACTIVITY NUMBER 21

Aim of the activity

To practise giving bad news.

The activity

The group breaks up into pairs and the pairs move to various parts of the room so that they are not immediately overheard by other pairs. In each pair, one person is nominated A and the other B. A then practises giving bad news to B, who responds according to the way that they experience that news being given. A should bear in mind the following three stages of breaking bad news:

1. a warning that bad news is coming, followed immediately by:
2. the bad news, itself, broken clearly and calmly followed by:
3. the teller of the news offering practical support.

Examples of 'bad news' that can be broken, include:

- the death of a relative,
- the news that the person's job has had to be terminated,
- failure of an examination.

After ten minutes, roles are reversed and B breaks bad news to A.

After a second ten minutes, the group reconvenes and group members discuss what happened during the activity. These comments may be jotted down onto a flip-chart sheet, white or blackboard, by the facilitator.

ACTIVITY NUMBER 22

Aim of the activity

Identify your style.

The activity

The group breaks up into pairs and the pairs move to various parts of the room so that they are not immediately overheard by other pairs. In each pair, one person is nominated A and the other B. Each pair then spends ten minutes identifying what they consider are their strengths and weaknesses in terms of being assertive or being submissive. Each pair identifies those situations that they can handle assertively and those situations that they cannot.

After ten minutes, the group reconvenes and group members discuss what happened during the activity. These comments may be jotted down onto a flip-chart sheet, white or blackboard, by the facilitator. The items identified during this activity may then be used as the basis of an assertiveness skills workshop. Role-play can be used to practise an assertive approach in those situations that most group members find difficult.

ACTIVITY NUMBER 23

Aim of the activity

To explore assertive behaviour through slow role-play.

The activity

The facilitator helps the group to identify a situation which most group members would find difficult to handle in terms of being assertive. She then sets up a role-play to explore the use of an assertive approach and group members are encouraged to act out the role-play with the central character practising assertive behaviour. The role-play should take place slowly and may be stopped at any time either by the central character or by other players in the role-play. It is stopped in order that a particular aspect may be 'replayed' and thus improved upon. The aim is to slowly build up a scenario in which assertive behaviour is demonstrated smoothly and effectively.

This exercise can be compared to rehearsing a play.

ACTIVITY NUMBER 24

Aim of the activity

To explore assertiveness in a group context.

The activity

The group remains in the circle and one person is invited to describe a situation in which they would like to have been assertive and were not. The person then describes the dialogue that occurred right up to the point when they failed to be assertive. e.g.

> A friend asked me to go to the theatre and I didn't really want to go. I thought I would tell him that I didn't want to and promised to go on another occasion. He then said he would be very disappointed if I didn't go, so I said ...'

Having stopped at this point, each person in the group is invited to offer an assertive response, in their own words. In this way a whole variety of perceived assertive statements is generated.

When each person has made a statement in response to the suggested scenario, the person who offered the scenario is invited to suggest which of the alternatives she feels would best have dealt with the situation.

ACTIVITY NUMBER 25

Aim of the activity

To explore psychodrama.

The activity

A member of the group is invited to recall a situation in which they would like to have been assertive but were not. She then describes the whole scenario to the group in some detail and identifies the other characters that were involved in the scenario.

The person then invites other members of the group to play the parts of the other characters involved in the original scenario. The scenario is then played out as it occurred, with occasional 'direction' from the person who suggested the scenario.

After this 'literal' run through, the group stops to discuss in what ways the person could have been more assertive in the playing out. A second run through then occurs. This time, the central player relives the scene but incorporates into her action the suggestions as to how she might be more assertive. In this way, the original scenario is replayed as an assertive scenario.

After this second run through, the group then discusses to what degree the 'assertive performance' was effective.

ACTIVITY NUMBER 26

Aim of the activity

To identify the behaviours that are associated with being assertive, being submissive and being aggressive.

The activity

The group breaks up into pairs and the pairs move to various parts of the room so that they are not immediately overheard by other pairs. In each pair, one person is nominated A and the other B.

Each pair is then given flip-chart sheets and asked to sketch caricatures of three people:

1. a submissive person,
2. an assertive person, and
3. an aggressive person.

After ten minutes, the group reconvenes and group members discuss what happened during the activity. The pairs pin up their sketches and other group members are encouraged to view these. Out of this viewing of the sketches can arise a discussion about the specific behaviours that are associated with the three different sorts of behaviours. These can be listed on flip-chart sheets by the facilitator.

Note: It is helpful (particularly for the less artistic!) if the group members are encouraged to draw large 'matchstick men' to serve as outlines for their 'people'. In this way, facial expressions and arm and leg positions can be drawn quite easily.

ACTIVITY NUMBER 27

Aim of the activity

To explore being assertive.

The activity

The group is simply asked to negotiate part of the day's (or week's) proceedings. The only 'ground rule' is that they should do this assertively and ensure that their needs and wants are catered for.

Following this period of negotiation, the group members are encouraged to discuss to what degree they felt they were :

- submissive,
- assertive, or
- aggressive.

ACTIVITY NUMBER 28

Aim of the activity

To set personal contracts.

The activity

The group breaks up into pairs and the pairs move to various parts of the room so that they are not immediately overheard by other pairs. In each pair, one person is nominated A and the other B. A then writes down a number of 'resolutions' that will serve as personal reminders about how she will be more assertive in the future. She then discusses these with her partner. After ten minutes, roles are swapped and B writes down her resolutions and discusses them with A. Table 8.1 is a useful format for noting these resolutions:

Table 8.1 Opportunities for, and constraints on, assertiveness

Situation in which I will be more assertive	What I will have to do to be more assertive in that situation	Possible constraints
1. (e.g. Saying 'no' to colleagues and friends)	(e.g. Control my anxiety; be prepared to repeat myself)	(e.g. Certain friends will push me to say 'yes'; some people may not like me as a result)
2.		
3.		
4.		

After ten minutes, the group reconvenes and group members discuss what happened during the activity. These comments may be jotted down onto a flip-chart sheet, white or blackboard by the facilitator. Group members are encouraged to talk through their resolutions with the group and to discuss the consequences of such resolutions.

ACTIVITY NUMBER 29

Aim of the activity

Assessment of strengths and weaknesses.

The activity

Group members are encouraged to 'brainstorm' activities that they feel represent awkward or difficult ones in terms of social skills. Examples, here, may be:

- entering a large room that is full of strangers;
- initiating a conversation at a party;
- introducing self to a stranger etc.

Having negotiated a short list of problem situations, group members are invited to jot down that list.

The group breaks up into pairs and the pairs move to various parts of the room so that they are not immediately overheard by other pairs. Each pair then spends ten minutes identifying what they consider are their strengths and weaknesses in those situations. Group members are encouraged to identify the specific behaviours that they would or would not find difficult to use.

After ten minutes, the group reconvenes and group members discuss what happened during the activity. These comments may be jotted down onto a flip-chart sheet, white or blackboard, by the facilitator. The items identified during this activity may then be used as the basis of a series of role-plays to practise the social skills that may be useful in these settings.

ACTIVITY NUMBER 30

Aim of the activity

Exploring poor social skills.

The activity

The group identifies a social situation that most people would find difficult to cope with. A role-play is then set up to explore this situation and the 'actors' in the role-play are invited to play their parts by demonstrating a total lack of social skills! This can be a dramatic method of identifying, paradoxically, the social skills that are required in a given situation. It can also highlight the sorts of everyday social skills problems that occur. In exaggerating poor social skills, 'normal' and everyday presentations of self are often highlighted!

After the role-play the group reconvenes and group members discuss what happened during the activity. These comments may be jotted down onto a flip-chart sheet, white or blackboard, by the facilitator. The items identified during this activity may then be used to practise 'proper' social skills.

ACTIVITY NUMBER 31

Aim of the activity

To assess other people's social skill levels.

The activity

The group breaks up into pairs and the pairs move to various parts of the room so that they are not immediately overheard by other pairs. In each pair, one person is nominated A and the other B. A then tells B what she considers to be that person's particular social skills. For example, she may say:

'I think that you handle group situations very well ... you are particularly good at putting people at their ease ...'

and so forth.

After ten minutes, roles are reversed and B then tells A what she considers to be that person's particular social skills.

After ten minutes, the group reconvenes and group members discuss what happened during the activity. These comments may be jotted down onto a flip-chart sheet, white or blackboard, by the facilitator. Out of this discussion can emerge the areas of social skills training for further work. This exercise is best carried out only with a group that is fairly mature and whose members know each other fairly well.

ACTIVITY NUMBER 32

Aim of the activity

Exploring critical incidents.

The activity

Group members are shown either:

1. a series of slides or
2. a short sequence of video film.

Each slide or sequence of film should graphically illustrate a difficult social situation. Examples for use here are:

- a person pushing into a queue of other people;
- a person who 'overtalks' in a conversation and doesn't allow the other person to leave the encounter;
- someone making an unwelcome sexual advance.

Where slides are used, the facilitator may have to 'talk through' the action represented in the slide. The aim of both slides or video tape should be that the situations act as 'triggers' for discussion.

After seeing each 'trigger', the group discusses ways that the social situation could best be dealt with. After that, a series of role-plays are set up and enacted to explore the various possibilities raised in the group discussion.

ACTIVITY NUMBER 33

Aim of the activity

Trying out new body language.

The activity

Participants break into pairs and spend ten minutes 'rearranging' the way each other is sitting. The person who is being rearranged should remain completely flexible and allow themselves to be moved into other positions. After ten minutes the pairs return to the larger group but each person remains in the new position and a discussion is held about the nature of body language.

ACTIVITY NUMBER 34

Aim of the activity

To explore the use of eye contact.

The activity

The group breaks up into pairs and the pairs move to various parts of the room so that they are not immediately overheard by other pairs. In each pair, one person is nominated A and the other B. A then talks to B, while B listens and makes constant and sustained eye contact! After ten minutes, roles are reversed, for a further ten minutes. Neither aspect of the pairs activity should evolve into a conversation. In the 'listening' role, the person just listens and makes sustained eye contact.

After ten minutes, the group reconvenes and group members discuss what happened during the activity. These comments may be jotted down onto a flip-chart sheet, white or blackboard by the facilitator. The group then discusses the uses and abuses of eye contact in therapeutic and everyday situations.

ACTIVITY NUMBER 35

Aim of the activity

To explore body posture, while listening.

The activity

Gerard Egan (1986) suggests that the following behaviours are usefully demonstrated while listening to another person in a therapeutic encounter.

1. Sit squarely in relation to the other person.
2. Maintain an 'open' position, with legs uncrossed and arms unfolded.
3. Lean slightly towards the other person.
4. Maintain reasonable eye contact.
5. Relax.

The group breaks up into pairs and the pairs move to various parts of the room so that they are not immediately overheard by other pairs. In each pair, one person is nominated A and the other B. A then talks to B for ten minutes while B listens but contradicts the first four behaviours identified above. Thus, B sits next to A, she crosses her legs and folds her arms, she leans away from the other person and she maintains no eye contact with the other person.

After ten minutes, roles are reversed and B talks to A while A contradicts the first four behaviours outlined above.

After a further ten minutes, the group reconvenes and group members discuss what happened during the activity. These comments may be jotted down onto a flip-chart sheet, white or blackboard, by the facilitator.

In the second stage of the activity, the whole process is repeated but this time each 'listener' in the pairs adopts the listening behaviours outlined by Egan. In the discussion that follows, Egan's behaviours are discussed as to their degree of appropriateness and effectiveness in therapeutic situations.

ACTIVITY NUMBER 36

Aim of the activity

To experience an absence of facilitation.

The activity

This group activity is simple to instigate if not to carry out! Group members remain in a circle and are told that there will be no facilitator for the session (about 45 minutes) and no subject for discussion. The group is left to its own devices.

After the 45 minutes has elapsed, group members and facilitator share their perceptions of the activity.

ACTIVITY NUMBER 37

Aim of the activity

To explore a directive style of group facilitation.

The activity

Group members remain in a circle and a volunteer from the group is invited to facilitate a group discussion for about 30 minutes.

The facilitator conducts the discussion using a directive style of facilitation. That is to say that she uses the following sorts of facilitative interventions:

- direct questions;
- summaries of what has been said;
- interventions which encourage each person in the group to speak;
- interventions which 'shut out' the overeager speaker, and so on.

At the end of the discussion the volunteer facilitator sums up what has been discussed.

At the end of the 30 minutes, a group discussion is held about the appropriateness or otherwise of the person's facilitation skills. Comments may be recorded on a flip-chart sheet or on the white or blackboard. A discussion is also held on the relative value of this style of interventions when compared to other styles described in this series of activities.

ACTIVITY NUMBER 38

Aim of the activity

To explore a non-directive style of group facilitation.

The activity

Group members remain in a circle and a volunteer from the group is invited to facilitate a group discussion for about 30 minutes.

The facilitator uses a non-directive style of group facilitation. She restricts herself to those interventions that encourage the development of discussion, such as:

- open-ended questions,
- reflections,
- empathy-building statements.

She makes no attempt to lead or direct the discussion in any way and makes no attempt to sum up what has been talked about at the end of the 30 minutes.

At the end of the 30 minutes, a group discussion is held about the appropriateness or otherwise of the person's facilitation skills. Comments may be recorded on a flip-chart sheet or on the white or blackboard. A discussion is also held on the relative value of this style of interventions when compared to other styles described in this series of activities.

ACTIVITY NUMBER 39

Aim of the activity

To explore an interpretative style of group facilitation.

The activity

Group members remain in a circle and a volunteer from the group is invited to facilitate a group discussion for about 30 minutes.

The volunteer facilitator uses an interpretative style of group leadership. Thus she may offer comments on what is happening within the group (the group process) or she may offer interpretations of what people are saying in the group (the group content). Interpretative frameworks used in this exercise will depend upon the group members' experience, education and belief system. She may, for example, offer interpretations from one or more of the following interpretative frameworks:

- psychodynamic,
- behavioural,
- symbolic interactionist,
- religious,
- sociological
- transactional analytical and so forth.

At the end of the 30 minutes, a group discussion is held about the appropriateness or otherwise of the person's facilitation skills. Comments may be recorded on a flip-chart sheet or on the white or blackboard. A discussion is also held on the relative value of this style of interventions when compared to other styles described in this series of activities.

ACTIVITY NUMBER 40

Aim of the activity

To explore a non-interpretative style of group facilitation.

The activity

Group members remain in a circle and a volunteer from the group is invited to facilitate a group discussion for about 30 minutes.

During the discussion, the facilitator encourages group members to offer interpretations of either what is happening within the group (the group process) or interpretations of what is being said in the group (the group content). She makes no interpretations herself of neither what is going on nor what is being said.

At the end of the 30 minutes, a group discussion is held about the appropriateness or otherwise of the person's facilitation skills. Comments may be recorded on a flip-chart sheet or on the white or blackboard. A discussion is also held on the relative value of this style of interventions when compared to other styles described in this series of activities.

ACTIVITY NUMBER 41

Aim of the activity

To explore a structured style of group facilitation.

The activity

Group members remain in a circle and a volunteer from the group is invited to facilitate a group discussion for about 30 minutes.

The facilitator offers the group a structured activity to carry out, that will take about 20 minutes to complete. Examples of such activities can be gleaned from the many titles that appear in the bibliography appending this book. The final ten minutes of the period is allowed for a free discussion of what happened during the structured activity.

At the end of the 30 minutes, a group discussion is held about the appropriateness or otherwise of the person's facilitation skills. Comments may be recorded on a flip-chart sheet or on the white or blackboard. A discussion is also held on the relative value of this style of interventions when compared to other styles described in this series of activities.

ACTIVITY NUMBER 42

Aim of the activity

To explore a unstructuring style of group facilitation.

The activity

Group members remain in a circle and a volunteer from the group is invited to facilitate a group discussion for about 30 minutes.

The facilitator suggests that the group decides how it would like to use the 30 minutes and makes no attempt to structure the time in any way at all. She does not attempt to draw up an agenda with the group, nor suggest a plan of action derived from what individual members suggest. She merely allows the group discussion to unfold and makes no attempt to structure it in any way. She may, of course, join in with the discussion but in no sense acts as a chairperson. Instead, she encourages the group to find its own way.

At the end of the 30 minutes, a group discussion is held about the appropriateness or otherwise of the person's facilitation skills. Comments may be recorded on a flip-chart sheet or on the white or black board. A discussion is also held on the relative value of this style of interventions when compared to other styles described in this series of activities.

ACTIVITY NUMBER 43

Aim of the activity

To explore a cathartic style of group facilitation.

The activity

This is an activity for a group that has had some training in handling the emotional release of others.

Group members remain in a circle and a volunteer from the group is invited to facilitate a group discussion for about 30 minutes.

The facilitator invokes a discussion around the topic of how people in the group are feeling. During the discussion, she invites anyone who is emotionally stirred by the discussion to allow themselves to express their feelings and to note any insights that such release may bring. A wide range of cathartic interventions may be used. For examples of such interventions, see Heron (1977b) and Burnard (1985).

At the end of the 30 minutes, a group discussion is held about the appropriateness or otherwise of the person's facilitation skills. Comments may be recorded on a flip-chart sheet or on the white or blackboard. A discussion is also held on the relative value of this style of interventions when compared to other styles described in this series of activities.

ACTIVITY NUMBER 44

Aim of the activity

To explore a non-cathartic style of group facilitation.

The activity

Group members remain in a circle and a volunteer from the group is invited to facilitate a group discussion for about 30 minutes.

The facilitator invokes a discussion on an emotive issue but does not encourage the free expression of emotion. Instead, she practises 'lightening' the atmosphere by the use of such interventions as:

- the use of humour,
- a change of topic,
- switching the discussion to another member of the group and so on.

At the end of the 30 minutes, a group discussion is held about the appropriateness or otherwise of the person's facilitation skills. Comments may be recorded on a flip-chart sheet or on the white or blackboard. A discussion is also held on the relative value of this style of interventions when compared to other styles described in this series of activities.

ACTIVITY NUMBER 45

Aim of the activity

To explore a disclosing style of group facilitation.

The activity

Group members remain in a circle and a volunteer from the group is invited to facilitate a group discussion for about 30 minutes.

The facilitator invites the group to join in a discussion on any topic and during that discussion, the facilitator offers her own points of view as an equal member of the group. She also allows herself to share something of how she is feeling with the group and thus 'personalizes' the discussion.

At the end of the 30 minutes, a group discussion is held about the appropriateness or otherwise of the person's facilitation skills. Comments may be recorded on a flip-chart sheet or on the white or blackboard. A discussion is also held on the relative value of this style of interventions when compared to other styles described in this series of activities.

ACTIVITY NUMBER 46

Aim of the activity

To explore a non-disclosing style of group facilitation.

The activity

Group members remain in a circle and a volunteer from the group is invited to facilitate a group discussion for about 30 minutes.

The facilitator invites the group to join in a discussion on any topic and during that discussion, the facilitator does not offer her own points of view on the topic under discussion. Neither does she share with the group how she is feeling. In this sense, she remains a 'blank' to the group.

It is arguable that if this exercise is being carried out as the first exercise that a particular group takes part in, then any observations that group members make about the facilitator will necessarily be 'projections' on the part of that group member. In other words, as the group member knows nothing about the group facilitator (because she is remaining 'non-disclosing'), then anything that another person says about her is likely to be actually true of that person himself!

At the end of the 30 minutes, a group discussion is held about the appropriateness or otherwise of the person's facilitation skills. Comments may be recorded on a flip-chart sheet or on the white or blackboard. A discussion is also held on the relative value of this style of interventions when compared to other styles described in this series of activities.

9 | Presentation skills training across organizations

Throughout the book, to this point, there has been an accent on teaching interpersonal skills to health professionals through getting students to reflect on their own skills, identify strengths and deficits, clarify what new skills need to be learned and through practising those new skills. The emphasis has also been on the importance of underlying values and beliefs in this process. The argument – and it is a pervasive one – is that behaviours, of themselves, are not enough. There must be something more 'behind' the behaviours. There is, however, another approach and that is simply to train people in a particular set of behaviours that are pre-determined by the organization. This is not to say, of course, that values and beliefs have somehow disappeared in this model: it is rather that the focus of those values and beliefs have shifted from the **individual** to the **health care organization**. There is a fine balance to be achieved, as Pennington notes well.

> Throughout our lives attempts are made, either directly or indirectly, to influence the way we think, feel and behave. Similarly, we spend much time in social interaction attempting to influence others to think, feel and act as we do. Indeed, the continuance of any society demands a degree of *conformity* to social norms; society also demands people to *comply* with requests and *obey* authority at times. However, people are not sheep, they do not blindly conform, comply or obey whenever the opportunity arises ... the individual is often placed in the conflicting situation of needing to maintain his or her own sense of identity and independence while at the same time being required or expected to conform, obey or comply with other people's wishes, prevailing norms, or standard. Failure to fall in with the 'crowd' may incur painful penalties ... failure to achieve and maintain a sense of identity may result in low self-esteem, low self-confidence and, in more extreme cases, depression and apathy (Pennington, 1986).

We must be careful, then, to keep an eye on the **individual** in the health care organization as well as keeping an eye on the corporate policy of that organization.

If we consider the behaviours that we see exhibited by staff in shops, in hotels and on airlines, we will see that they offer a consistent – if some would say 'artificial' – set of behaviours. Whether or not those behaviours **are** construed as artificial is a moot point. One may, for example, want to argue, simply, that those are the behaviours that go with the role. If you work in a hotel, then it is expected that you will offer a certain level of 'presentation of self' to the customer. In the health care professions, however, there has been a certain reluctance to adopt this point of view. It is raised in this chapter simply to expand the debate, to explore alternatives and to propose the question: 'is a fairly rudimentary training in certain "standard" presentation behaviours better than no training at all?' And the supplementary question: 'should we aim at ensuring that **everyone** in any given health care setting can deliver a certain level of presentation?' If the answer to either or both of these questions is 'no', then we need to return to the model so far described in this book and focus, almost exclusively on the 'individual values and beliefs drive the behaviours' argument. If the answer is a tentative 'yes' to either or both of these questions, then we need to consider training methods.

It does seem likely that given the emphasis on quality and the assessment of quality, that every element of the health care service – either private or public – will come under increasing scrutiny. This is bound to include the assessment of how well or how badly staff greet and work with the public. In this sense, then, it is reasonable to argue that we should at least consider some methods of training people in baseline presentational skills. It seems to me that there may be various 'levels' of training in this field and these are best illustrated in Figure 9.1.

We will notice, then, that while almost **everyone** in a health care organization might be trained in stage one skills, only a very few might be trained in stage three skills. And, in a sense, this probably echoes the general situation that

Stage one skills	Basic presentation skills for all staff working in health care arenas.
Stage two skills	'Advanced' training for those who offer a particular 'caring' role: nurses, doctors, etc.
Stage three skills	Specific training in counselling or psychotherapy for those whose primary work is in one of these fields.

Figure 9.1 Three levels of interpersonal skills training in a health care organization

is in place at the moment. All that this simple model does is to **formalize** the situation and to offer a framework for developing things further.

The **way** in which such skills training is introduced needs to be considered. There is a tendency for a single, highly motivated manager – who is convinced of the need for change within an organization – to want to try to change the organization, single-handed. Georgiades and Phillimore (1975), in an important paper, called these sorts of people 'hero-innovators' and warn:

> The idea [is] that you can produce, by training, a knight in shining armour who, loins girded with new technology and beliefs, will assault his organisational fortress and institute changes both in himself and others at a stroke. Such a view is ingenuous. The fact of the matter is that organisations such as schools or hospitals will, like dragons, eat hero-innovators for breakfast.

In place of the 'hero-innovator', Georgiades and Phillimore suggest six positive guidelines for introducing change into an organization and these will apply to the introduction, across an organization, of presentational skills of the sort discussed in this chapter.

1. Try to work with those supportive forces within the organization, rather than against those who are resistant to change.
2. Aim to produce a self-motivated team of workers who are powered from within themselves.
3. Work with the 'healthy' parts of the system, i.e. those who have the motivation and resources to be improved, rather than on lost causes.
4. Ensure that the people you are working with for change have the freedom and authority to implement the proposed changes.
5. Try to obtain involvement of key personnel in the change programme, but make this realistic and appropriate.
6. Protect team members from undue stress and pressure (Georgiades and Phillimore, 1975).

The whole issue of how presentational skills training in any given organization is introduced needs careful consideration. Some people in the organization will have been doing an excellent job for many years and may resent the idea of their having to 'practise' or 'relearn' new skills. There are others who will resent the idea because it will mean change itself. Others will object to the notion of an 'across the organization' policy on interpersonal communication and are likely to see it as 'artificial' or false. The possibility of introducing such change needs, then, to be 'sold' to the organization's members and must be promoted as a good thing for everyone: for the patients, clients and customers **and** for the staff themselves. How this is achieved, locally, will depend on the management structures in place in various organizations. There is evidence, though, that the **worst** way to try to implement change is simply to force it on an organization. Much negotation and discussion needs to take place if organization members are to be convinced of the need to formalize a policy on inter-personal communication and much compromise may also be needed. Indeed, in the ideal situation, perhaps, the organization **itself** identifies the appropriate behaviours that are required by the staff – perhaps through focus groups and small work groups.

We might argue that stage two and three skills have been dealt with, already, in this book. The skills of the nurse, doctor or occupational therapist (and these are only examples – there are many other health care workers who work directly with patients) are ones that might be developed through the experiential learn-ing methods described in this book. We might ask those professionals, during their training, to reflect on what they do in order to enhance their skills. We might also use experiential learning methods to develop stage three skills. Most counsellors and therapists are trained either in small groups or by **being** in counselling or therapy themselves and thus learning 'experientially' anyway.

The gap, it seems to me, is in straightforward methods in dealing with stage one skills and this chapter considers some ways in which this deficit might be met.

First, we need to consider the parameters of the task. I suggest that we need to consider, at least, the following issues:

- large numbers of staff are likely to require training;
- training methods need to be effective but 'non-invasive'; many of the staff involved in such training may not want to 'explore themselves' in any depth but may simply want to pick up what are seen to be the appropriate presenta-tion skills for their functioning in the organization;
- there need to be ways of assessing people's skills and maintaining their qual-ity.

The issue of large numbers is an increasing one in higher education. As health care training moves directly into the higher education sector, the increase in student numbers becomes more acute. As we have seen from other chapters in this book, many ideas in interpersonal skills training depend on the intimacy of small group work. With larger groups, however, the need to **plan** and **struc-ture** group activities carefully becomes more evident. It is probably true to say that **process** issues in groups becomes less important as the groups get larger. With larger groups it is no longer possible for any given trainer or facilitator to pay close attention to what individuals are doing and feeling.

Second, we need to consider what sort of skills might be considered under the heading of 'presentation skills'. I would suggest that these might include at least the following:

- introducing self to clients, consumers and customers;
- answering the telephone and dealing with enquiries;
- dealing with questions;
- giving basic information and advice;

- dealing with complaints;
- offering an 'approachable' and pleasant manner that projects a positive image of self and of the health care organization.

The list could, of course, be added to. My aim is simply to point to some of the basic interpersonal skills that might be useful to a very wide range of people in any given health care organization, from administrative staff to social workers and from cleaners to psychiatrists. In a sense, many of the skills are probably little more than a reminder of what some would claim to be 'good manners' in dealing with the public.

A MODEL FOR TRAINING IN PRESENTATION SKILLS

The model offered here is a tentative one and one that draws on many of the principles so far discussed. The model is, however, rather more **prescriptive** than is the case with the 'fully experiential' approach. It does not lean so heavily on seeking the views of participants but offers, instead, rather more explicit guidelines about how to proceed. Figure 9.2 illustrates the six stages in the proposed model.

	Goal	Achieved by
Stage one	Identification of the core presentation behaviours required by the health care organization	The health care organizations' training team
Stage two	Preparation of video film of the behaviours or training of trainers in demonstrating 'excellent' examples	The health care organizations' training team or by a third-party company
Stage three	Demonstration of the behaviours to employees in the health care organization	The training team
Stage four	Practice, through guided role-play and coaching, by the employees	The training team
Stage five	Assessment of employees' presentation skills in the training situation and then in the 'real' situation	The training team and by participants
Stage six	Monitoring of staff performance, including the maintenance of quality assurance procedures	All members of the organization

Figure 9.2 A model for training in presentation skills

STAGE ONE: IDENTIFICATION OF THE CORE PRESENTATIONAL BEHAVIOURS

In this stage, through various levels of consultation within the health care organization, a policy is devised for what are felt to be the 'best' presentation skills that might be used by all staff within that organization. Such consultation might include dicussion with consultants, managers, educators and trainers both inside and outside the organization. The initial brainstorming sessions within this stage are likely to highlight various differences of opinion and should also produce stimulating debate. The process does, however, need to be carefully chaired in order for the planning team to reach its objective: the clear identification of certain core skills. These skills must then be broken down into **microskills** in order that they be taught.

The interpersonal skills audit

In line with other quality assurance methods, one way of identifying the sorts of interpersonal skills that are required for effective health care delivery in any given organization is to perform an interpersonal skills audit. In an earlier chapter, we saw how Heron's Six Category Intervention Analysis could be used in interpersonal skills training (Heron, 1986). It can also be used as part of an interpersonal skills audit. In this case, a designated health care manager either interviews staff or observes the sorts of interpersonal skills being regularly used within the service. A template can be devised for noting the sorts of skills being used and Figure 9.3 is an example of such a template. Using this template, the auditor identifies frequently used skills throughout the organization and, in this way, builds up a profile of the sorts of skills that need to be taught to practitioners joining the organization.

STAGE TWO: PREPARATION OF TRAINING MATERIALS

The next stage involves the preparation of training material. This is likely to involve the preparation of video tapes illustrating exemplars of good presentation skills. It is good practice to make these tapes as professional as possible to ensure their credibility. To that end, it may be worthwhile (and worth the considerable financial investment) to employ professional audio-visual experts in the making of such a tape. Tapes can also be used to illustrate **bad** as well as good practice.

An alternative (or perhaps accompaniment) to the use of video tape presentation is the skilled demonstration of the required skills by trainers. If this is done, then the trainers (usally a pair or a small team) need to rehearse the skills so that their performance is as flawless as possible. It also takes confidence to stand up in front of a group and claim a certain level of presentational expertise.

Type of intervention	Notes	Examples of interpersonal skills
Prescriptive	Clients are often given instructions about timing of appointments	Clear and unambiguous statements, followed by support
Informative	Clients are regularly offered advice about various Acts of Parliament relating to their situation	Clearly given information
Confronting	Spouses are often challenged about their behaviour in relation to the client and her family	Challenging statements
Cathartic	Practitioners frequently encourage clients to express their feelings about the situations in which they find themselves	Support through the discharge of emotion
Catalytic	Practitioners often encourage clients to elaborate on their situations through the use of open-ended questions and reflection of thoughts and feelings	Questions, reflection, empathy building statements
Supportive	Practitioners often assure clients that the health care facility is available to them at any time	Offers of support. Validating statements

Figure 9.3 Template for noting skills

STAGE THREE: DEMONSTRATION OF THE BEHAVIOURS

In the third stage, a short lecture or discussion on the need for quality interpersonal behaviour and on how it might be achieved is offered. This can be augemented by handouts that reinforce the lecture. Then, short excerpts of tape are played to illustrate particular microskills. Alternatively, as we have seen, trainers demonstrate those microskills. This stage needs to be followed up fairly quickly with **practice** so that the exemplars offered are still in the minds of the participants in the session.

STAGE FOUR: PRACTICE THROUGH ROLE-PLAY

In stage four, the participants pair off and role-play the various microskills. During these role-plays, the trainers act as **coaches** in a specific way. The trainer sits with the person role-playing a particular piece of behaviour and encourages the performance and offers minor or major suggestions about changes to the performance. In this way, the trainer operates in much the same was as the director of a play. The point is, also, to correct 'mistakes' as quickly as possible so that a good, skilled performance is achieved as quickly as possible. On the other hand, participants are also 'allowed' to make mistakes and there does not have to be any sense of competition in the training area.

After each set of role-plays, participants should be encouraged to discuss what they have achieved in a open group discussion, facilitated by the trainers. The focus of these discussions should be on how the skills can be transferred into the 'real' situation.

It is important, too, that as the various microskills are rehearsed, they are also brought together into 'complete performances'. For example, if the skill of working through the process of introducing yourself to a small group of other people is broken down into small stages, the **whole** process of the introduction should also be practised.

What is also vital is that at the end of each training session, participants must be encouraged to **use** their skills as quickly as possible after the session.

STAGE FIVE: ASSESSMENT

At the end of each microskills training activity, an assessment of skills should be carried out. This can be done either by one of the trainers or by one of the participants in the group who has been briefed to carry out the assessment. Such assessment should offer the participant who has been role-playing information about the following:

- the level of skill demonstrated;
- what needs to be improved;
- what was done well;
- any other comments on performance.

At the end of each training session, there should also be an **evaluation** of the day's work during which participants offer a comment, each, about what they **least** liked about the day and what they **most** liked about it. Trainers may also invite evaluative comments about **their** performance. At the end of the training course, the trainers should have prepared a more formal evaluation questionnaire.

STAGE SIX: MONITORING

The most important thing of all is that the presentation skills learned during the training exercises are carried over into the real situation of day to day health care. This can partly be achieved through all managers and trainers helping to develop a culture in which attention is paid, at all times, to self-presentation. They should also be prepared to **role-play** excellent presentation skills every day as part of their own work. They should also be prepared to offer prompt and positive feedback on 'good' performance as they see it. There will necessarily be a 'run in' period where people are adjusting to using their new skills and follow-up, reinforcement workshops are likely to be necessary. In the end, though, staff members also have to become self-monitoring and reflective on their own interpersonal processes. This can be aided by trainers holding a thorough discussion on these topics during the training sessions. Staff members do, of course, have to **want** to achieve a high level of interpersonal competence. Internal motivation is, in the end, the most powerful sort.

There must be also a frequent seeking of the patient or clients' opinions about the level of interpersonal skill being offered and this should be part of the health care organization's quality audit procedure. However, it seems unlikely that simple, pen and paper questionnaires will get to the **heart** of effective interpersonal performance and it is to be hoped that quality managers will also make sure that a percentage of patients or clients are invited to be **interviewed** about their care. In turn, those quality managers will also have to be skilled in sensitive interviewing and, themselves, show high levels of interpersonal competence.

Finally, there is a constant need to ensure that quality issues are squarely addressed. Not only must an audit trail be maintained – a process by which each element of training is recorded and in which all assessments and evaluations are recorded – but consumers must be polled for their views of how well staff are performing. The data obtained from that polling must be fed back into the system and appropriate changes made to the training system to ensure a high-quality service.

DISCUSSION

This chapter has offered a very much shorter version of interpersonal skills training than has been offered in other parts of the book. However, all of the main **principles** described elsewhere in the book can be applied in this approach. The main differences between what has gone before and what is contained in this chapter is the amount of **control** the facilitator or trainer has over the **content** of the training. In this approach, it is taken for granted that the health care organization will have a large say in the form and style of the basic skills to be displayed by employees. This raises a number of questions. First, we might ask whether or not managers – or educators – are the best arbiters of what does and what does not constitute effective interpersonal behaviour. As has been suggested, it may be useful, here, to bring in outside consultants. It seems likely that such an exercise might be a 'one-off' activity. Once base line skills are defined and described, then such skills may be used for a reasonable amount of time in training workshops with only minimal changes. However, the initial stage of describing and defining a wide range of microskills is likely to be time consuming and, potentially, expensive.

The second point is that it seems likely that there will be some casualties in this approach – people who, for whatever reason – cannot be 'trained' into offering a particular style or level of interpersonal behaviour. This causes something of a dilemma that could, perhaps, only be resolved on a local, policy-making basis. Do you, on the one hand, stipulate that all employees within an organization **must** reach a certain level of performance (or leave that organization) or do you allow some 'slack' in the system that would enable individuals some degree of 'interpretation' of the standards? This is a complicated issue. On the one hand, it seems important that high interpersonal standards are maintained at all times. On the other, it seems less than desirable to have an organization run by people who are merely acting out a set of prescribed behaviours in a mechanical way. Certainly, as people progress from stage one skills (above) to stage two and stage three skills, it seems likely that a greater amount of latitude will be essential to allow for professional judgement and contextual circumstances.

To some, this approach may seem mechanistic, driven by financial considerations and even politically expedient. It may reflect, however, a changing view of how some people view the role of health care workers in the later part of the twentieth century. The accent, recently, has been much more on quality assurance in all parts of the health care service – both public and private. Also, much more attention is paid to how all types of services are delivered to consumers – both within and outside of the health care arena. It might be naive to suggest that all of the basic training of health care workers can be left to chance – that basic interpersonal skills might be learned 'on the job'. When that happens, some people do pick up the skills while others do not. This method, at the very least, ensures that all of the people within an organization are made aware of their interpersonal performance and given a chance to reflect on it. The most crucial issue, perhaps, is how the organization responds to those members of the staff who **adapt** the behaviours to any great degree. Health care is not the same as the 'care' offered by hotel or catering staff. Health care workers are not dealing, simply, with consumers but with people who find themselves in difficult, often painful and often frightening situations. Clearly, this type of interpersonal training, **on its own**, is not enough. Such training must also be backed up by discussions about care, about psychology, sociology, health care policy and all of the other topics that are included in most modern syllabi. The **degree** to which these other topics are included in training programmes might vary with the **roles** of the people involved. It might be reasonable to offer only the bones of the training described here to certain staff, while others – and particularly those who have direct dealings with patients or clients – be offered more advanced training and education.

The approach advocated in this chapter also assumes that the trainers involved will be skilful. Role-playing and coaching of the type described here involves a considerable degree of awareness and expertise on the part of the trainers. This is not something to be taken on lightly. Rather, if an organization decides to pursue this path of 'quality interpersonal presentation', then that organization must be prepared to make the necessary investment in the training of the trainers. Many colleges and university departments and many private organizations now offer facilitator trainings of various sorts.

AN EXAMPLE IN PRACTICE: A CASE STUDY

Life is usually more complicated than it is portrayed in books. All sorts of practical, organizational and political factors mitigate against the smooth implementation of theory into practice. The following is an example of how one health care institution planned and implemented the training of a large group of health care students in interpersonal skills. It will become evident that **some** of the principles discussed in this chapter and in this book were implemented while other factors also played a part.

Stage one: the workgroup

The first stage was for the head of curriculum development in the college to form a small working group to discuss the training of the health care students. This consisted of five interested people: a clinical psychologist, an interpersonal skills trainer and two practising clinicians. The group discussed a range of possible ways of introducing interpersonal skills training into a central degree course in the college. It was acknowledged that, given the number of students involved, the course could only be run over a single year of the course. This, in itself, would involve 120 students. It was agreed that an interpersonal skills training course could not be **lecture**-based but would involve the development of a range of experiential workshops.

Finances were limited and it was appreciated that facilitators for the experiential workshops could not be 'brought in' to the college but would have to be found within it. To this end, it was agreed that the curriculum organizer would poll all of the teaching staff of the college in order to find 15 interested lecturers who would be prepared to train as 'facilitators' of groups of eight students. It was also appreciated that there was little 'slack' time in the students' timetable and the most teaching time that could be found was eight sessions of one hour, distributed throughout the academic year. In practice, this meant that the workshops would be held once a month throughout the second year of the course.

Initially, it was difficult to find 15 people who were either a) interested in acting as facilitators or b) would admit to having the time to work in this way. Eventually, after an open meeting and after all staff in the college had acknowledged that interpersonal skills training was now a **requirement** in the curriculum, 15 people were recruited. This 15 was made up mostly of lecturers within the college but those lecturers were also supplemented by 'buying in' some help from freelance trainers.

Training the trainers

Once the group of facilitators was formed, a series of 'training the trainers' meetings was held to train up the facilitators. These were organized by the original members of the workgroup. The workgroup met and agreed a programme of training that included the following points:

- how to run group discussions;
- how to use interpersonal skills exercises;
- how to deal with contingencies;
- how to evaluate and assess the course.

These training groups were run over a period of six months with participants meeting twice a month. Many of the sessions involved potential facilitators 'trying out' various exercises and activities in order to anticipate how they would 'work' with students. Probably because the group was self-selected and because motivation was high, the workshops and the training the trainers course generally went well and only one member left the group – and this was because of a promotion to another, more administrative, post. The member who left was replaced by another 'outside' trainer. At the end of the six month period, most of the trainee facilitors felt reasonably confident that they could run groups with students. At this time, too, a timetable for the eight sessions was worked out, as follows:

- Meeting 1: Introductory lecture to whole student group on 'Interpersonal Skills in Health Care';
- Meeting 2: Introductory lecture to whole student group on how the smaller workshops are to be organized;
- Meeting 3: First small workshop: self-presentation and introductions (i.e. becoming aware of the need to monitor 'self' and to pay attention to how students introduce themselves to clients);
- Meeting 4: Second small workshop: Taking a history (i.e. how the students conduct an exploratory interview with clients);
- Meeting 5: Discussing health care issues with clients;
- Meeting 6: Listening and responding (exercises in assessing students listening and questioning skills);
- Meeting 7: Dealing with problem situations (students invited to explore their own 'difficult' situations with clients through role-play);
- Meeting 8: Assessment and evaluation of course.

Running the workshops

The introductory lectures were given by two of the members of the workgroup – both of whom had had considerable experience of running communication and counselling courses. In the second lecture, students were given full details of how the subsequent meetings would be organized. Students were allocated to small groups and given a course book that offered full details of the course and a detailed booklist.

Attendance at the small group meeting was compulsory and the course was assessed and 'marks' generated which counted towards the students' degree classification. Self, peer and facilitator assessment was implemented.

Support groups were also implemented for the facilitators and these were also well attended. Most agreed that they enjoyed running the small groups and were able to draw on their considerable experience 'in the field' – in clinical settings. They also found that the small group work 'brought to life' their teaching and made a considerable and pleasant change to more 'formal' teaching – most of which, up to that point, had been lecturing.

During the small group workshops, various practical and interpersonal issues were discussed and worked through. All students were reminded of the need to make interpersonal skills part of their 'real life' experience in their day-to-day clinical work and this was reinforced by short, reflective sessions at the beginning of each of the meetings. For the first few minutes of each session, students were encouraged to discuss the interpersonal encounters they had experienced during the previous month. As might be expected, some students entered into the workshops wholeheartedly while others saw attendance as a necessary means of completing their course.

This, then, was one short example of how interpersonal skills training was implemented in one college in a health care setting. It was by no means a perfect course, nor was it the ideal length and depth. As with many things in education, compromises had to be made. The net result, however, was to make 'interpersonal skills' more of a central focus of the course in question. At the time of writing, plans are being put into practice to lengthen the course and to offer a more formal 'training the trainers' course.

One of the larger issues in the implementation of the programme is the **cultural** change that still has to occur in the organization. As we have seen in this chapter, the issue of changing the culture of an organization is a difficult one. In the college described here, there was – initially – considerable resistance in some quarters to the idea of interpersonal skills training being introduced at all. A number of the more senior members of the college felt that communication and interpersonal skills were 'already being taught' or 'did not need to be taught'. Role models of communication skills were not always exemplary but very senior staff could not be encouraged to reflect on their own skills. Clearly, the idea that **all** staff might review their interpersonal skills was professionally – as well as personally – threatening. It was appreciated (both at the beginning of the programme and throughout its implementation) that there needed to be **two** foci of attention:

- on training students in interpersonal skills and

- on attempting to modify the culture of the organization to make communication and interpersonal skills a high priority.

As might be imagined, the second issue proved to be the most difficult to address and it may be the case that a 'new generation' of health care students has to work through the system before real organizational changes are possible. As we have noted, real life situations are rarely perfect and often involve compromise. That has certainly been the case in the situation described here.

| 10 | **Conclusion** |

This book has described a range of theoretical and practical issues to do with teaching and learning interpersonal skills as they relate to the health professions. As a way of drawing together those ideas, the following is a checklist of issues that summarize many of the points made in the book.

- Keep things **simple**. It is easy to try to discuss or teach too many skills at once or to assume that everyone in a group needs to do 'something more advanced'. Most people can benefit from further practice in listening and responding. Make sure that the basics are covered before you move onto more 'complicated' skills. Usually, the simple ones are complicated enough anyway.

- Keep things **structured**. In the informal atmosphere that often arises out of interpersonal skills training groups it is often possible to be drawn into loose, unstructured discussions that take up valuable training time. Although discussion **is** important (and it is particularly important to allow plenty of time for 'processing' training exercises), also remember that you are involved in an **educational** enterprise. Use the time carefully.

- Keep a clear distinction between **education** and **therapy**. Although the distinction is not always a simple one, it is usually true to say that a trainer's contractual obligations towards her students are **educational**. You are not there to offer therapy. If the discussion heads towards very deep emotional areas, make sure of the following: (a) that you have had 'permission' from the group to explore issues like this, (b) that you have the skills to manage the situation and (c) you are completely clear in your own mind that what is happening is 'appropriate' to the setting. If in doubt, steer away from the therapeutic and keep things focussed on the educational.

- Allow plenty of time. This is a corollary of the point made above. The important 'learning time' in the use of experiential learning exercises often occurs during the discussion **after** the exercises. Make sure that you have allowed sufficient time for a full discussion to occur.

- Keep the atmosphere 'light'. Do not attempt to create a 'deep and meaningful' atmosphere in your workshop or training sessions. This can be off-putting for some participants and can lead to 'non-disclosure' in others – it can cause some people to 'shut down'. The lighter atmosphere is the one in which people can talk easily and discuss even the more difficult issues easily. A lot of this will depend on your own confidence as a trainer and on your own personality.

- Keep yourself fresh. It is easy to get drawn into running the same workshops and using the same activities over and over again. This can lead to what I call 'experiential burnout' – a state in which you feel unable to do any further facilitation because of either boredom with the approach or a feeling of having done the same thing too many times. Read some more books and attend some refresher workshops as a participant. Try new things. Change your programme a little, next time.

- Allow your participants choice, but don't make **every** issue a question of choice. On the one hand, you should be prepared to consult the group about major decisions (such as when you feel the need to change the course of a workshop) but you don't need to consult on everything. Very little gets done if you are constantly checking even the most basic issues with the group (e.g. 'Shall we break for coffee now, or later?' 'Shall we have 15 minutes or half an hour?' 'Shall we stay in this room or move to the larger one?'). Strike a balance between consulting the group and taking responsibility for some of the decisions yourself.

- Remember the voluntary principles. Do not force anyone to take part in a training exercise against their will. They may do the exercise but it is unlikely that they will learn anything very positive from it.

- Take plenty of breaks. The breaks in between training sessions are useful consolidation sessions. In them, participants try out new behaviours and even new language and ways of describing things. Also, experiential learning sessions can be tiring. Allow people some 'recovery time'.

- Stay open to criticism. Allow participants to challenge you and to disagree with you. You are not there to force on them a particular point of view. Facilitation also means facilitating disagreement.

- Try using lectures sometimes. Not everything can or needs to be taught experientially. Sometimes, a good 'theory' lecture can help to explain the background to a series of activities.

- Keep up your own education. None of us has ever finished our education. Be prepared to change your views and be prepared for these changes in view to affect your behaviour. You may well come to challenge the views expressed in books such as this one and that is no bad thing at all!

- Read the research. Experiential learning training has depended, until recently, on a considerable amount of **theory** but not a great deal of research. It is important that (a) more research into the field is carried out and (b) practitioners using experiential learning methods read and use that research.

- Develop your own style. In a sense, this is inevitable. A pattern that is followed by many people (and often seems to work) is that they begin by adopting another facilitator's style of working. After a while, through experience and practice, this becomes personalized and modified to suit that particular person's way of working.
- Evaluate what you do and invite evaluation. Be constructively critical of what you do and continue to invite feedback from your participants. Also consider joint facilitating groups and invite your co-facilitator to comment on your work. Be prepared to change as a result of what is said.

References

Alberti, R. E. and Emmons, M. L. (1982) *Your Perfect Right: A Guide to Assertive Living*, San Luis Obispo, California: Impact.

Aptekar, H. H. (1955) *The Dynamics of Casework and Counselling*, Cambridge, Mass.: Houghton Mifflin.

Argyle, M. (1975) *The Psychology of Interpersonal Behaviour*, Harmondsworth: Penguin.

Argyris, C. (1982) *Reasoning, Learning and Action*, San Francisco: Jossey Bass.

askSam Systems (1994) *askSam: The Database for Information*, Perry, Florida: askSam Systems.

Atwood, A. H. (1979) The mentor in clinical practice, *Nursing Outlook* **27**, 714–17.

Bailey, C. R. (1983) Experiential learning and the curriculum, *Nursing Times*, 20 July, 45–6.

Bandler, R. and Grinder, J. (1975) *The Structure of Magic: Volume I: A Book About Language and Therapy*, California: Science and Behaviour Books.

Banyard, P. and Hayes, N. (1994) *Psychology: Theory and Applications*, London: Chapman & Hall.

Basescu, S. (1990) Show and tell: Reflections on the analyst's self-disclosure. In G. Stricker and M. Fisher (eds), *Self-disclosure in the Therapeutic Relationship*, New York: Plenum Press.

Bateson, C. D. and Coke, J. S. (1981) Empathy: a source of altruistic motivation for helping? In J. P. Rushton and R. M. Sorventino, *Altruism and Helping Behaviour: Social, Personality and Developmental Perspectives*, New Jersey: Lawrence Erlbaum Associates.

Blackwell Software (1993) *Idealist for Windows*, Oxford: Blackwell Scientific Publications.

Blake, R. and Mouton, J. (1972) The D/D matrix : scientific methods. Cited in J. Heron (1975) *Six Category Intervention Analysis: Human Potential Research Project*, Guildford: University of Surrey.

Blaney, J. (1974) Program development and curricula authority. In J. Blaney, I. Housego and G. McIntoxh (eds), *Program Development in Education*, Vancouver: Centre for Continuing Education, University of British Columbia.

Bodley, D. E. (1992) Clinical supervision in psychiatric nursing: using the process recording, *Nurse Education Today*, **12**(2), 148–55

Bond, M. (1986) *Stress and Self-Awareness: A Guide for Nurses*, London: Heinemann.

Bond, M. and Kilty, J. (1986) *Practical Methods of Dealing with Stress*, 2nd edn, Human Potential Research Project, Guildford: University of Surrey.

Boreham. N. C. (1987) Learning from experience in diagnostic problem solving. In J. T. Richardson, M. W. Eysenck and D. W. Piper (eds), *Student Learning*, Milton Keynes: Open University Press.

Boud, D. (ed.)(1973) *Experiential Learning Techniques in Higher Education*, Human Potential Learning Project, Guildford: University of Surrey.

Boud, D., Keogh, R. and Walker, D. (1985) *Reflection: Turning Experience into Learning*, London: Kogan Page.

Boydel, T. (1976) *Experiential Learning*, Manchester Monograph No. 5, Manchester: Department of Adult and Higher Education, University of Manchester.

Brandes, D. and Phillips, R. (1984) *The Gamester's Handbook*, Vol. 2, London: Hutchinson.

Breese, J. (1983) Counselling pupils in centres for disruptives, *Maladjustment and Therapeutic Education* **1**(1), 6–12.

British Association for Counselling (BAC) (1989a) *Invitation to Membership*, Rugby: BAC.

British Association for Counselling (BAC) (1989b) *Code of Ethics and Practice for Counselling Skills*, Rugby: BAC.

Brodkey, H. (1995) *Profane Friendship*, London: Vintage.

Brookfield, S. D. (1986) *Understanding and Facilitating Adult Learning: A Comprehensive Analysis of Principles and Effective Practices*, Milton Keynes: Open University Press.

Brookfield, S. D. (1987) *Developing Critical Thinkers: Challenging Adults to Explore Alternative Ways of Thinking and Acting*, Milton Keynes: Open University Press.

Buber, M. (1948) *Tales of Hasidism: The Later Masters*, New York: Schocken.

Buber, M. (1958) *I and Thou*, 2nd edn, New York: Scribner.

Buber, M. (1966) *The Knowledge of Man: A Philosophy of the Interhuman*, ed. M. Friedman, trans. R. G. Smith, New York: Harper & Row.

Bullock, A. and Stallybrass, O. (1977) *The Fontana Dictionary of Modern Thought*, London: Fontana/Collins.

Burnard, P. (1985) *Learning Human Skills: A Guide for Nurses*, London: Heinemann.

Burnard, P. (1987a) Self and peer assessment, *Senior Nurse* **6**(5), 16–17.

Burnard, P. (1987b) *A Study of the Ways in Which Experiential Learning Methods Are Used to Develop Interpersonal Skills in Nurses in Canada and the United States*, London: National Florence Nightingale Memorial Committee.

Burnard, P. (1988) Experiential learning: some theoretical considerations, *International Journal of Lifelong Education* **7**(2), 127-33.

Burnard, P. (1989) *Counselling Skills for Health Professionals*, London: Chapman & Hall.

Burnard, P. (1990) *Learning Human Skills: An Experiential Guide for Nurses*, 2nd edn, Oxford: Butterworth-Heinemann.

Burnard, P. (1991) A method of analysing interview transcripts in qualitative research, *Nurse Education Today* **11**, 461–66.

Burnard, P. (1992a) *Experiential Learning in Action*, Aldershot: Avebury.

Burnard, P. (1992b) The free form database program as a research tool. *Nurse Education Today* **12**, 51–6.

Burnard, P. (1992c) Some problems in understanding other people: analysing talk in research, counselling and psychotherapy. *Nurse Education Today* **12**, 130–6.

Burnard, P. (1994) *Counselling Skills for Health Professionals*, 2nd edn, London: Chapman & Hall.

Burnard, P. and Morrison, P. (1988) Nurses' perceptions of their interpersonal skills: a descriptive study using Six Category Intervention Analysis, *Nurse Education Today* **8**, 266–72.

Burnard, P. and Morrison, P. (1989) What is an interpersonally skilled person?: A repertory grid account of professional nurses' views, *Nurse Education Today* **9**(6), 384–91.

Burton, A. (1977) The mentoring dynamic in the therapuetic transformation, *American Journal of Psychoanalysis* **37**, 115–22.

Callner, D. and Ross, S. (1978) The assessment and training of assertiveness skills with drug addicts: a preliminary study, *International Journal of the Addictions* **13**(2), 227–30.

Campbell, A. (1984) *Paid to Care?*, London: SPCK.

Clarke, B. and Feltham, W. (1990) Facilitating peer group teaching within nurse education, *Nurse Education Today* **10**, 54–7.

Cohen-Cole, S. A. and Bird, J. (1991) Function 1: gathering data to understand the patient. In S. A. Cohen-Cole (ed.), *The Medical Interview: the Three-Function Approach*, St Louis, Missouri: Mosby Year Book.

Coleman, J. S. (1976) Differences between experiential learning and classroom learning. In M. T. Keeton and Associates (eds), *Experiential Learning*, Washington, DC: Jossey Bass.

Collins, G. C. and Scott, P. (1979) Everyone who makes it has a mentor, *Harvard Business Review* **56**, 89–101.

Conrad, J. (1902, 1973) *Heart of Darkness*, Harmondsworth: Penguin.

Costello, J. (1989) Learning from each other: peer teaching and learning in student nurse training, *Nurse Education Today* **9**, 203—6.

Crompton, M. (1992) *Children and Counselling*, London: Edward Arnold.

Darling, L. A. W. (1984) What do nurses want in a mentor?, *Journal of Nursing Administration*, October, 42–4.

Dewey, J. (1916, 1966) *Democracy and Education*, London: Free Press.

Dewey, J. (1938, 1971) *Experience and Education*, London: Collier Macmillan.

Edelstein, B and Eisler, R. (1976) Effects of modelling and modeling with instruction and feedback on the behavioural components of social skills, *Behaviour Therapy* **4**, 382–9.

Egan, G. (1990) *The Skilled Helper: A Systematic Approach to Effective Helping*, 4th edn, Pacific Grove, California: Brooks/Cole.

Ellis, R. and Watson, C. (1987) Experiential learning: the development of communication skills in a group therapy setting, *Journal of Advanced Nursing* **7**, 215–21.

Ellis R. and Whittington, D. (1981) *A Guide to Social Skill Training*, London: Croom Helm.

FEU (1983) *Curriculum Opportunity: A Map of Experiential Learning in Entry Requirements to Higher and further Education Award Bearing Courses*, London: Further Education Unit.

Falloon, I., Lindley, P., Mcdonald, R. and Marks, I. (1977) Social skills training of out patient groups, *British Journal of Psychiatry* **131**, 599–609.

Fay, A. (1978) *Making Things Better By Making Them Worse*, New York: Hawthorne.

Fay, P. P. and Doyle, A. G. (1992) Stages of group development. In J. W. Pfeiffer and L. D. Goodstein (eds), *The 1982 Annual for Facilitators, Trainers and Consultants*, San Diego, California: University Associates.

Frankl, V. E. (1969) *The Will to Meaning*, New York: World Publishing Co.

Frankl, V. E. (1975a) Paradoxical intention and dereflection: a logotherapuetic technique, *Psychotherapy: Theory, Research and Practice* **12**(3), 226–37.

Frankl, V. E. (1975b) *The Unconscious God*, New York: Simon & Schuster.

Freire, P. (1972a) *Cultural Action for Freedom*, Harmondsworth: Penguin.

Freire, P. (1972b) *Pedagogy of the Oppressed*, Harmondsworth: Penguin.

French, P. (1994) *Social Skills for Nursing Practice*, 2nd edn, London: Chapman & Hall.

Gendlin, E. T. and Beebe, J. (1968) An experiential approach to group therapy, *Journal of Research and Developments in Education* **1**, 19–29.

Georgiades, N. and Phillimore, L. (1975) The myth of the hero-innovator and alternative strategies for organisational change. In C. Kierman and E. Woodford (eds), *Behaviour Modification with the Severely Mentally Retarded*, Amsterdam: Associated Scientific Publishers.

Gray, S. (1985) *Swimming to Cambodia: The Collected Works of Spalding Gray*, London: Picador.

Gross, R. (1977) *The Lifelong Learner*, New York: Simon & Schuster.

Grossman, R. (1985) Some Reflections on Abraham Maslow, *Journal of Humanistic Psychology* **25**(4), 31–4.

Hall, C. (1954) *A Primer of Freudian Psychology*, New York: Mentor Books.

Halmos, P. (1965) *The Faith of the Counsellors*, London: Constable.

Hampden-Turner, C. (1966) An existential learning theory, *Journal of Applied Behavioural Science* **12**(4).

Hanks, L, Belliston, L. and Edwards, D. (1977) *Design Yourself*, Los Altos, California: Kaufman.

Hargie, O., Saunders, C. and Dickson, D. (1981) *Social Skills in Interpersonal Communication*, 2nd edn, London: Croom Helm.

Heidegger, M. (1927, 1962) *Being and Time*, New York: Harper & Row.

Heron, J. (1970) *The Phenomenology of the Gaze*, Human Potential Research Project, Guildford: University of Surrey.

Heron, J. (1973) *Experiential Training Techniques*, Human Potential Research Project, Guildford: University of Surrey.

Heron, J. (1977a) *Behaviour Analysis in Education and Training*, Human Potential Research Project, Guildford: University of Surrey.

Heron, J. (1977b) *Catharsis in Human Development*, Human Potential Research Project, Guildford: University of Surrey.

Heron, J. (1981) Philosophical basis for a new paradigm. In P. Reason and J. Rowan, *Human Inquiry: A Sourcebook of New Paradigm Research*, Chichester: Wiley.

Heron J. (1982) *Education of the Affect*, Human Potential Research Project, Guildford: University of Surrey.

Heron, J. (1989) *The Facilitator's Manual*, London: Kogan Page.

Heron, J. (1990) *The Facilitators' Handbook*, London: Kogan Page.

Heron, J. (1986) *Six Category Intervention Analysis*, 2nd edn, Human Potential Research Project, Guildford: University of Surrey.

Hewitt, J. (1977) *Meditation*, Sevenoaks, Kent: Hodder & Stoughton.

Hobbs, T. (1992) Skills of communication and counselling. In T. Hobbs, *Experiential Training: Practical Guidelines*, London: Routledge.

Holmes, J. and Lindley, R. (1991) *The Values of Psychotherapy*, Oxford: Oxford University Press.

Hough, M. (1994) *A Practical Approach to Counselling*, London: Pitman Publishing.

Hovand, D. and Janis, I. (1959) *Personality and Persuadability*, New Haven, Connecticut: Yale University Press.

Hovand, D., Janis, I. and Kelley, H. (1953) *Communications and Persuasion*, New Haven, Connecticut: Yale University Press.

Husserl, E. (1931) *Ideas: General Introduction to Pure Phenomenology*, trans G. Boyce, London: Allen & Unwin.

Infante, M. S. (1986) The conflicting roles of nurse and nurse educator. *Nursing Outlook* **34**(2), 94–6.

Janis, I. (ed.) (1982) *Counselling on Personal Decisions*, New Haven, Connecticut: Yale University Press.

Jarvis, P. (1983) *Professional Education*, London: Croom Helm.

Jarvis, P. (1987) *Adult Learning in the Social Context*, London: Croom Helm.

Jenkins, E. (1987) *Facilitating Self-Awareness, A Learning Package Combining Group work with Computer Assisted Learning*, Wigan: Open Software Library.

Johns, G. and Morris, N. (1988) Nursing hopes, *Open Mind* **30**, 16—17.

Jones, A. (1994) *Counselling Adolescents, School and After*, London: Kogan Page.

Jourard, S. (1964) *The Transparent Self*, Princeton, New Jersey: Van Nostrand.

Jourard, S. (1971) *Self-Disclosure: an Experimental Analysis of the Transparent Self*, Chichester: Wiley.

Kalisch, B. J. (1971) Strategies for developing nurse empathy, *Nursing Outlook* **19**(11), 714–17.

Keeton, M. and Associates (1976) *Experiential Learning*, San Francisco, California: Jossey Bass.

Kelly, G. (1955) *The Psychology of Personal Constructs*, 2 vols, New York: Norton.

Kelly, G. (1969) The autobiography of a theory. In B. Maher, *Clinical Psychology and Personality: The Selected Papers of George Kelly*, New York: Wiley.

Kelly, G. A. (1970) A brief introduction to personal construct theory. In D. Bannister, *Perspectives in Construct Theory*, New York: Academic Press.

Kilty, J. (1978) *Self and Peer Assessment*, Human Potential Research Project, Guildford: University of Surrey.

Kilty, J. (1982) *Experiential Learning*, Human Potential Research Project, Guildford: University of Surrey,

Kilty, J. (1987) *Staff Development for Nurse Education: Practitioners Supporting Students*. A Report of a 5-Day Development Workshop, Human Potential Research Project, Guildford: University of Surrey.

King, E. C. (1984) *Affective Education in Nursing: A Guide to Teaching and Assessment*, Maryland: Aspen.

King-Spooner, S. (1995) Psychotherapy and the white dodo, *Changes* **13**(1), 45–51.

Kirschenbaum, H. (1979) *On Becoming Carl Rogers*, New York: Dell.

Knowles, M. (1975) *Self Directed Learning*, New York: Cambridge Books.

Knowles, M. (1980) *The Modern Practice of Adult Education: From Pedagogy to Andragogy*, 2nd edn, Chicago: Follett.

Knowles, M. (1990) *The Adult Learner: A Neglected Species*, 4th edn, Houston, Texas: Gulf.

Knowles M. and Associates (1984) *Andragogy in Action: Applying Modern Principles of Adult Learning*, San Francisco, California: Jossey Bass.

Koberg, D. and Bagnall, J. (1981) *The Revised All New Universal Traveler: A Soft-Systems Guide to Creativity, Problem-Solving and the Process of Reaching Goals*, Los Altos, California: Kaufmann.

Kolb, D. (1984) *Experiential Learning*, Englewood Cliffs, New Lawton: Prentice Hall.

Lawton, D. (1973) *Social Change, Educational Theory and Curriculum Planning*, London: Hodder & Stoughton.

Lindeman, E. (1956) The democratic man. In R. Gessner (ed.), *Selected Writings*, Boston: Beacon Press.

Lindeman, E. C. (1926) *The Meaning of Adult Education*, New York: New Republic.

LoBiondo-Wood, G. and Haber, J. (1994) *Nursing Research: Methods, Critical Appraisal and Utilization*, 3rd edn, St Louis: Mosby.

Luft, J. (1969) *Of Human Interaction*, The Johari Model, Palo Alto, California: Mayfield.

Lundsteen, S. (1971) *Listening: Its Impact on Reading and Other Language Acts*, New York: National Council for Teachers of English.

MacDonald, J. (1992) Project 2000 curriculum evaluation: the case for teacher evaluation. *Nurse Education Today* **12**(2), 101–7.

Macquarrie, J. (1973) *Existentialism*, Harmondsworth: Penguin.

Mallon, B. ((1987) *An Introduction to Counselling Skills for Special Educational Needs*, Manchester: Manchester University Press.

Maslow, A. (1972) *Motivation and Personality*, 2nd edn, New York: Harper & Row.

May, K. M. *et al.* (1982) Mentorship for scholarliness: opportunities and dilemmas, *Nursing Outlook* **30**, 22–8.

May, T. (1993) *Social Research: Issues, Methods and Processes*, Milton Keynes: Open University Press.

Meyeroff, M. (1972) *On Caring*, New York: Harper & Row.

Michelson, L., Sugari, D., Wood, R. and Kazadin, A. (1983) *Social Skills Assessment and Training with Children*, New York: Plenum Press.

Miles, M. B. and Huberman, A. M. (1994) *Qualitative Data Analysis*, London: Sage.

Mocker, D. W. and Spear, G. E. (1982) *Lifelong Learning: Formal, Non-formal and Self-Directed*, The ERIC Clearinghouse on Adult Career and Vocational Education, Ohio: Columbus.

Moreno, J. L. (1959) *Psychodrama*, Vol. II, Beacon, New York: Beacon House Press.

Moreno, J. L. (1969) *Psychodrama*, Vol. III, Beacon, New York: Beacon House Press.

Moreno, J. L. (1977) *Psychodrama*, Vol. I, 4th edn, Beacon, New York: Beacon House Press.

Morris, D. (1977) *Manwatching: A Field Guide to Human Behaviour*, London: Triad/Panther.

Morrison, P. (1994) *Caring for Patients*, London: Baillière Tindall.

Moustakas, C. (1994) *Phenomenological Research Methods*, Thousand Oaks, California: Sage.

Murgatroyd, S. (1982) Experiential learning and the person in pursuit of psychology, *Education Section Review (British Psychological Society)* **6**(2), 112–17.

Murgatroyd, S. (1986) *Counselling and Helping*, Methuen, London

Naranjo, C. and Ornstein, R. E. (1971) *On the Psychology of Meditation*, London: Allen & Unwin.

Nelson-Jones, R. (1981) *The Theory and Practice of Counselling Psychology*, London: Holt Rinehart & Winston.

Nelson-Jones, R. (1995) *The Theory and Practice of Counselling*, 2nd edn, London: Cassell.

Newble, D. and Cannon, R. (1987) *A Handbook for Medical Teachers*, 2nd edn, Lancaster: MTP Press.

Newell, R. (1994) *Interviewing Skills for Nurses and Other Health Care Professionals: A Structured Approach*, London: Routledge.

Noonan, E. (1983) *Counselling Young People*, London: Methuen.

Open University Coping With Crisis Group (1987) *Running Workshops: A Guide for Trainers in the Helping Professions*, London: Croom Helm.

Ouspensky, P. D. (1988) *Conscience: The Search for Truth*, London: Arkana.

Packham, R., Roberts, R. and Bawden, R. (1989) Our faculty goes experiential. In S. Warner Weil and I. McGill (eds), *Making Sense of Experiential Learning*, Milton Keynes: Open University.

Patton, M. Q. (1982) *Practical Evaluation*, Beverly Hills, California: Sage.

Pennington, D. C. (1986) *Essential Social Psychology*, London: Edward Arnold.

Peters. R. S. (1969) *Ethics and Education*, London: Allen & Unwin.

Peters, R. S. (1972) Education as initiation. In R. D. Archambault (ed.), *Philosophical Analysis and Education*, London: Routledge & Kegan Paul.

Pfeiffer, J. W. and Goodstein, L. D. (1982) *The 1982 Annual for Facilitators, Trainers and Consultants*, San Diego, California: University Associates.

Pfeiffer, J. W. and Jones, J. E. (1974 and ongoing) *A Handbook of Structured Experiences for Human Relations Training*, Vol. 2, La Jolla, California: University Associates.

Pirsig. R. (1974) *Zen and the Art of Motor Cycle Maintenance*, London: Arrow.

Polyani, M. (1958) *Personal Knowledge*, Chicago: University of Chicago Press.

Postman, N. and Weingartner, C. W. (1969) *Teaching as a Subversive Activity*, Harmondsworth: Penguin.

Pring, R. (1976) *Knowledge and Schooling*, London: Open Books.

Quinn, F. M. (1995) *The Principles and Practice of Nurse Education*, 3rd edn, London: Chapman & Hall.

Reber, A. (1985) *The Penguin Dictionary of Psychology*, Harmondsworth: Penguin.

Redwine, M. (1989) The autobiography as a motivational factor for students. In S. Warner Weill and I. McGill (eds), *Making Sense of Experiential Learning*, Milton Keynes: Open University.

Riebel, L. (1984) A homeopathic model of psychotherapy, *Journal of Humanistic Psychology* **24**(1), 9–48.

Robinson, K. and Vaughan, B. (1992) *Knowledge for Nursing Practice*, Oxford: Butterworth-Heinemann.

Rogers, C. R. (1951) *Client-Centred Therapy*, London: Constable.

Rogers, C. R. (1957) The necessary and sufficient conditions of therapeutic personality change, *Journal of Consulting Psychology* **21**, 95–104.

Rogers, C. R. (1967) *On Becoming a Person*, London: Constable.

Rogers, C. R. (1972) The facilitation of significant learning. In M. L. Silberman, J. S. Allender and J. M. Yanoff, *The Psychology of Open Teaching and Learning: An Inquiry Approach*, Boston, Mass.: Little, Brown & Co.

Rogers, C. R. (1983) *Freedom to Learn for the Eighties*, Columbus: Merrill.

Rogers, C. R. (1985) Toward a more human science of the person, *Journal of Humanistic Psychology* 25(4), 7–24,

Rogers, C. R. and Stevens, B. (1967) *Person to Person: The Problem of Being Human*, Lafayette, California: Real People Press.

Rosenberg, M. and Hovand, C. (eds)(1960) *Attitude, Organization and Change*, New Haven, Connecticut: Yale University Press.

Rowan, J. (1983) *The Reality Game: A Guide to Humanistic Counselling and Therapy*, London: Routledge.

Rowe, D. (1990) Introduction. In J. Masson, *Against Therapy*, London: Fontana.

Ryle, G. (1949) *The Concept of Mind*, Harmondsworth: Peregrine.

Sarantakos, S. (1993) *Social Research*, Basingstoke: Macmillan.

Sartre, J-P. (1956) *Being and Nothingness*, New York: Philosophical Library.

Schön, D. A. (1983) *The Reflective Practitioner: How Professionals Think in Action*, London: Temple Smith.

Schulman, E. D. (1982) *Intervention in Human Services: A Guide to Skills and Knowledge*, 3rd edn, St Louis, Missouri: C.V. Mosby.

Scriven, M. (1967) The methodology of evaluation. In R. W. Tyler (ed.), *Perspectives in Curriculum Evaluation*, Chicago: Rand McNally.

Searle, J. R. (1983) *Intentionality: An Essay in Philosophy of the Mind*, Cambridge: Cambridge University Press.

Self, W. (1994) *My Idea of Fun*, Harmondsworth: Penguin.

Skilbeck, M. (1984) *School Based Curriculum Development*, London: Harper & Row.

Steil, L. (1991) Listening training: the key to success in today's organizations. In D. Borisoff and M. Purdy (eds), *Listening in Everyday Life*, Maryland: University of America Press.

Sundeed, S. J., Stuart, G. W., Rankin, E. D and Cohen, S. A. (1989) *Nurse-Client Interaction: Implementing the Nursing Process*, St Louis: Mosby.

Trower, P. (ed.) (1984) *Radical Approaches to Social Skills Training*, London: Croom Helm.

Tuckman, B. W. (1965) Development sequence in small groups, *Psychological Bulletin* 63(6).

Vonnegut, K. (1967) *Mother Night*, London: Cape.

Vonnegut, K. (1983) *Deadeye Dick*, London: Panther.

Weil, S. W. and McGill, I. (eds)(1989) *Making Sense of Experiential Learning*, Milton Keynes: Open University Press.

Whitehead, A. N. (1933) *The Aims of Education*, London: Benn.

Whorf, B. J. (1956) *Language, Thought and Reality: Selected Writings*, Cambridge, Mass.: Technology Press of Massachusetts Institute of Technology.

Woolfe (eds) *Handbook of Counselling in Britain*, London: Tavistock/Routledge.

Woolfe, R. (1992) Experiential learning in workshops. In T. Hobbs (ed.), *Experiential Training: Practical Guidelines*, London: Routledge.

Woolfe, R., Dryden, W. and Charles-Edwards, D. (1989) The nature and range of counselling practice. In W. Dryden, D. Charles-Edwards and R. Woolfe (eds), *Handbook of Counselling in Britain*, London: Routledge.

Zuker, E. (1983) *Mastering Assertiveness Skills*, New York: American Management Association.

Further reading

This bibliography should help you to find other works on the themes discussed in this book. Entries that can be considered as 'essential reading' are preceded by an asterisk, to make the list more user-friendly.

Abbey, D. S., Hunt, D. E. and Weiser, J. C. (1985) Variations on a theme by Kolb: a perspective for understanding counselling and supervision. *Counselling Psychologist* **13**, 477–501.

Abrami, P., Leenthal, L. and Perry, R. (1982) Educational seduction, *Review of Educational Research* **52**, 446–64.

Adkins, W. R. (1984) Life skills education: a video-based counselling/learning delivery system. In D. Larson (ed.), *Teaching Psychological Skills: Models for Giving Psychology Away*, Pacific Grove, CA: Brooks/Cole.

Allan, D. M. E., Grosswald, S. J. and Means, R. P. (1984) Facilitating self-directed learning. In J. S. Green, S. J. Grosswald, E. Suter and D. B. Walthall (eds), *Continuing Education for the Health Professions: Developing, Managing and Evaluating Programs for Maximum Impact on Patient Care*, San Francisco, California: Jossey Bass.

Allcock, N. (1992) Teaching the skills of assessment through the use of an experiential workshop, *Nurse Education Today*, **12**(4), 287–92.

Altshuler, K. Z. (1989) Will the psychotherapies yield different results? A look at assumptions in therapy trials, *American Journal of Psychotherapy* **63**(3), 310–20.

Anderson, B. and Anderson, W. (1985) Client perceptions of counselors using positive and negative self-involving statements, *Journal of Counselling Psychology* **32**, 462–5.

Anderson, M. and Gerrard, B. (1984) A comprehensive interpersonal skills program for nurses, *Journal of Nursing Education*, **23**(8), 353–5.

Aniouwu, E. (1991) A multi-ethnic approach ... a community genetic counselling course ... focus on four genetic conditions, *Nursing (London) The Journal of Clinical Practice Education and Management*.

Argyle, M. (ed.) (1981) *Social Skills and Health*, London: Methuen.

Argyle, M. (1988) *Bodily Communication*, London: Routledge.

Argyris, C. (1982) *Reasoning, Learning and Action*, San Francisco: Jossey Bass.

Arnold, E. and Boggs, K. (1989) *Interpersonal Relationships: Professional Communication Skills for Nurses*, Philadelphia, PA: Saunders.

Ashworth, P. D. and Longmate, M. A. (1993) Theory and practice: beyond the dichotomy, *Nurse Education Today* 13(5), 321–7.

Atkins, S. and Murphy, K. (1993) Critical thinking: a foundation for consumer-focused care, *Journal of Continuing Education in Nursing* 18(8), 1188–92.

Austin, E. K. (1981) *Guidelines for the Development of Continuing Education Offerings for Nurses*, Norwalk, Connecticut: Appleton-Century-Crofts,

Bachelor, A. (1988) How clients perceive therapist empathy: a content analysis of 'received' empathy, *Psychotherapy* 25, 277–40.

Barkham, M. J. and Shapiro, D. A. (1986) Counsellor verbal response modes and experienced empathy, *Journal of Counselling Psychology* 33(1), 3–10.

Barkham, M. J. and Shapiro, D. A. (1990) Exploratory therapy in two-plus-one sessions: a research model for studying the process of change. In G. Lietaer, J. Rombouts and R. Van Balen (eds), *Client-centered and Experiential Psychotherapy in the Nineties*, Leuven: Leuven University Press, 429–46.

Barkham, M., Shapiro, D.A. and Firth-Cozens, J. (1989) Personal questionnaire changes in prescriptive vs. exploratory psychotherapy, *British Journal of Clinical Psychology* 28, 97–107.

Barrett-Lennard, G. T. (1981) The empathy cycle – refinement of a nuclear concept, *Journal of Counselling Psychology* 28, 91–100.

Baruth, L. G. (1987) *An Introduction to the Counselling Profession*, Englewood Cliffs, NJ: Prentice-Hall.

Bass, B. M. (1981) *Stogdill's Handbook of Leadership*, New York: Free Press.

Bayntun, Lees D. (1993) Setting the scene for experiential learning, *Nursing Standard* 7(36), 28–30.

Belkin, G. S. (1987) *Contemporary Psychotherapies*, 2nd edn, Pacific Grove, CA: Brooks/Cole.

Benjamin, A. (1981) *The Helping Interview*, 3rd edn, Boston: Houghton Mifflin.

Berger, D. M. (1984) On the way to empathic understanding, *American Journal of Psychotherapy* 38, 111–20.

Binder, J. L. (1993) Observations on the training of therapists in time-limited dynamic psychotherapy, *Psychotherapy* 30(4), 592–8.

Bohart, A. C. (1988) Empathy: client-centred and psychoanalytic, *American Psychologist* 43, 667–8.

Bolton, E. B. (1980) A conceptual analysis of the mentoring relationship in the career development of women, *Adult Education* 30, 195–207.

Bond, T. (1993) *Standards and Ethics for Counselling in Action*, London: Sage.

Boone, E. J., Shearon, R. W., White, E. E. and Associates (1980) *Serving Personal and Community Needs Through Adult Education*, San Francisco, California: Jossey Bass.

Bor, R. and Watts, M. (1993) Talking to patients about sexual matters, *British Journal of Nursing* **2**(13), 657–61.

Botkin, J., Elmandjra, M. and Malitza, M. (1979) *No Limits to Learning: Bridging the Human Gap*, London: Pergamon.

*Boud, D., Keogh, R. and Walker, M. (1985) *Reflection: Turning Experience into Learning*, London: Kogan Page.

*Boud, D. J. (ed.) (1981) *Developing Student Autonomy in Learning*, London: Kogan Page.

Bower, G. H. and Hilgard, E. R. (1981) *Theories of Learning*, 5th edn, Englewood Cliffs, NJ: Prentice Hall.

*Bowling, A. (1991) *Measuring Health: A Review of Quality of Life Scales*, Milton Keynes: Open University Press.

Boydel, E. M. and Fales, A. W. (1983) Reflective learning: key to learning from experience, *Journal of Humanistic Psychology* **23**(2), 99–117.

Bozarth, J. D. (1984) Beyond reflection: emergent modes of empathy. In R. Levant and J. Shlien (eds), *Client-Centred Therapy and the Person-Centered Approach: New Directions in Theory, Research and Practice*, New York: Praeger, 59–75.

Brammer, L. M. (1988) *The Helping Relationship: Process and Skills*, Englewood Cliffs, NJ: Prentice Hall.

Brammer, L. M., Shrostrom, E. and Abrego, P. (1988) *Therapeutic Psychology: Fundamentals of Counselling and Psychotherapy*, Englewood Cliffs, NJ: Prentice Hall.

Brandon, D. (1991) Counselling mentally ill people, *Nursing Standard* **6**(7), 32–3.

Brown, D. and Srebalus, D. J. (1988) *An Introduction to the Counselling Process*, Philadelphia, PA: Prentice Hall.

Brown, J. E. and Slee, P. T. (1986) Paradoxical strategies: the ethics of intervention, *Professional Psychology: Research and Practice* **17**, 487–91.

Bruckner-Gordon, F., Gangi, B. K. and Wallman, G. U. (1988) *Making Therapy Work*, New York: Harper & Row.

Brundage, D. H. and Mackeracher, D. (1980) *Adult Learning Principles and their Application to Program Planning*, Ontario: Ministry of Education.

Buchan, R. (1991) An integrated model of counselling, *Senior Nurse* **11**(4), 32–3.

Buckroyd, J. and Smith, E. (1990) Learning to help ... teaching counselling, *Nursing Times* **86**(35), 54–7.

Budman, S. H. and Gurman, A. S. (1988) *Theory and Practice of Brief Therapy*, New York: Guilford Press.

Burke, J. F. (1989) Contemporary approaches to psychotherapy and counselling: the self-regulation and maturity model, *Pacific Grove*, CA: Brooks/Cole.

Byrne, S. (1991) Counselling – and essential nursing skill, *World of Irish Nursing* **20**(4), 26–7.

Cameron, B. L. and Mitchell, A. M. (1993) Reflective peer journals: developing authentic nurses, *Journal of Advanced Nursing* **18**(2), 290–7.

*Carkhuff, R. R. (1969a) *Helping and Human Relations: Vol. 1. Selection and Training*, New York: Holt, Rinehart & Winston.

*Carkhuff, R. R. (1969b) *Helping and Human Relations: Vol. 2. Practice and Research*, New York: Holt, Rinehart & Winston.

Carkhuff, R. R. (1971a) *The Development of Human Resources*, New York: Holt, Rinehart & Winston.

Carkhuff, R. R. (1971b) Training as a preferred mode of treatment, *Journal of Counselling Psychology* **18**, 123–31.

Carkhuff, R. R. (1985) *PPD: Productive Program Development*, Amherst, MA: Human Resource Development Press.

Carkhuff, R. R. (1987) *The Art of Helping*, 6th edn, Amherst, MA: Human Resource Development Press.

Carpio, B. A. and Majumdar, B. (1993) Experiential learning: an approach to transcultural education for nursing, *Journal of Transcultural Nursing*, **4**(2), Winter, 4–11.

Carty, E. M., Conine, T. A. and Hall, L. (1990) Comprehensive health promotion for the pregnant woman who is disabled: the role of the midwife, *Journal of Nurse Midwifery*, **353**, 133–42.

Clark, D. (1991) Guidance, counselling therapy: responses to 'marital problems' 1950–90, *The Sociological Review* **39**, 765–98.

Clark, J. M., Hopper, L. and Jesson, A. (1991) Communication skills: progression to counselling, *Nursing Times* **87**(8), 41–3.

Clarke, L. (1989) Intervention and certainty in counselling literature Part 1, *Senior Nurse* **9**(4), 18–19

Clawson, J. G. (1985) Is mentoring necessary?, *Training and Devlopment Journal* **39**(4), 36–9.

Clift, I. and Magee, T. (1992) Developing a new counselling course, *Nursing Standard* **6**(18), 34–6.

Clift, J. C. and Imrie, B. W. (1981) *Assessing Students and Appraising Teaching*, London: Croom Helm.

Clutterbuck, D. (1985) *Everybody Needs a Mentor: How to Further Talent Within an Organisation*, London: The Institute of Personnel Management.

Collins, N. W. (1983) *Professional Women and Their Mentors*, Englewood Cliffs, NJ: Prentice Hall.

Combs, A. W. (1986) What makes a good helper? A person-centred approach, *Person-Centered Review* **1**, 51–61.

Confer, W. N. (1987) *Intuitive Psychotherapy: The Role of Creative Therapeutic Intervention*, New York: Human Sciences Press.

Conyne, R. K. (1987) *Primary preventive counselling*, Muncie, Indiana: Accelerated Development.

Corey, G., Corey, M. S. and Callanan, P. (1988) *Issues and Ethics in the Helping Professions*, 3rd edn, Pacific Grove, CA: Brooks/Cole.

Cormier, L. S. (1987) *The Professional Counsellor: A Process Guide to Helping*, Englewood Cliffs, NJ: Prentice Hall.

Corsini, R. and Wedding, D. (1989) *Current Psychotherapies*, 4th edn, Itasca, IL: F.E. Peacock.

Cox, M. (1978) *Structuring the Therapuetic Process: Compromise With Chaos*, Oxford: Pergamon.

Cramer, D. (1992) *Personality and Psychotherapy: Theory, Practice and Research*, Buckingham: Open University Press.

Crandall, S. (1993) How expert clinical educators teach what they know, *Journal of Continuing Education in the Health Professions*, **13**(1), 85–98.

Crits-Christoph, P., Baranackie, K. and Kurcias, J. (1991) Meta-analysis of therapist effects in psychotherapy outcome studies, *Psychological Testing*, 3rd edn, New York: Harper & Row.

Cross, K. P. (1981) *Adults as Learners*, San Francisco: Jossey Bass.

Cross-Durrant, A. (1984) Lifelong education in the writings of John Dewey, *International Journal of Lifelong Education* **3**(2), 115–25.

Crute, V. C. *et al.* (1989) An evaluation of a communication skills course for health visitor students, *Journal of Advanced Nursing* **14**(7), July, 546–52.

Curtis, T. and Kibler, S. (1990) Counselling in cancer care, *Nursing Times* **86**(51), 25–7.

Daly, M. J. and Burton, R. L. (1983) Self-esteem and irrational beliefs: an exploratory investigation with implications for counselling, *Journal of Counselling Psychology* **30**, 361–6.

Darbyshire, P. (1993) In the hall of mirrors ... reflective practice, *Nursing Times* **89**(49), 26–9.

Darkenwald, G. G. and Merriam, S. B. (1982) *Adult Education: Foundations of Practice*, New York: Harper & Row.

Davies, J. M. (1991) A behavioural model for counselling the nursing mother, *Breastfeeding Review* **2**(4), 154–7.

Davison, J. (1992) Approach with care ... Individual or group counselling, *Nursing Times* **88**(8), 38–9.

*Debord, J. B. (1989) Paradoxical interventions: a review of the recent literature, *Journal of Counselling and Development* **67**, 394—98.

Denelsky, G. Y. and Boat, B. W. (1986) A coping skills model of psychological diagnosis and treatment, *Professional Psychology: Research and Practice* **17**, 322–30.

Denton, P. L. (1992) Teaching interpersonal skills with videotape ... to chronically ill psychiatric clients, *Occupational Therapy in Mental Health* **2**(4), 17–34.

Derlega, V. J. and Berg, J. H. (1987) *Self-disclosure: Theory, Research, and Therapy*, New York: Plenum.

Dewing, J. (1990) Reflective practice ... within primary nursing from individual and group viewpoints, *Senior Nurse*, **10**(10), 26–8.

*Dickson, A. (1985) *A Woman in Your Own Right: Assertiveness and You*, London: Quartet Books.

Dillon, J. T. (1990) *The Practice of Questioning*, London: Routledge.

Dimmock, B. (1992) A child of our own ... frequency and intensity of problems about pregnancy and young children in stepfamilies, *Health Visitor* **65**(10), 368–70.

Dobson, K. S. and Shaw, B. F. (1993) The training of cognitive therapists: what have we learned from treatment manuals?, *Psychotherapy* **30**(4), 573–7.

Docking, S. (1994) Accredited learning – the assessment procedure: how to complete the assessment for the reflective practice module, *Professional Nurse* **9**(4), 244–6.

Donley, R. J., Horan, J. J. and DeShong, R. L. (1989) The effect of several self-disclosure permutations on counselling process and outcome, *Journal of Counselling and Development* **67**, 408–12.

Dorn, F. J. (1984) *Counselling as Applied Social Psychology: An Introduction to the Social Influence Model*, Springfield, IL: Charles C. Thomas.

Dryden, W. and Ellis, A. (1986) Rational-emotive therapy. In W. Dryden and W. L. Golden (eds), *Cognitive-behavioural Approaches to Psychotherapy*, London: Harper & Row.

*Dryden, W. and Trower, P. (eds) (1988) *Developments in Cognitive Psychotherapy*, Newbury Park, CA: Sage Publications.

Dryden, W. and Yankura, J. (1992) *Daring to be Myself*, Buckingham: Open University Press.

Dubrin, A. J. (1987) *The Last Straw: How to Benefit from Trigger Events in Your Life*, Springfield, IL: Charles C. Thomas.

Duncan, S. and Fiske, D. W. (1977) *Face-to-Face Interaction: Research, Methods and Theory*, Hillsdale, New Jersey: Lawrence Erlbaum Associates.

Eisenberg, N. and Strayer, J. (eds) (1987) *Empathy and Its Development*, New York: Cambridge University Press.

Elias, J. L. and Merriam, S. (1980) *Philosophical Foundations of Adult Education*, Florida: Krieger.

Elliott, R. (1986) Interpersonal Process Recall (IPR) as a psychotherapy process research method. In L. S. Greenberg and W. M. Pinsof (eds), *The Psychotherapeutic Process: A Research Handbook*, New York: Guilford Press, 249–86.

Elliott, R. and James E. (1989) Varieties of client experience in psychotherapy: an analysis of the literature, *Clinical Psychology Review*, **9**, 443–67.

Elliott, R. and Shapiro, D. A. (1992) Client and therapist as analysts of significant events. In S. G. Toukmanian and D. L. Rennie (eds), *Psychotherapy Process Research: Paradigmatic and Narrative Approaches*, London: Sage, 163–86.

Ellis, A. (1983) How to deal with your most difficult client: you, *Journal of Rational-Emotive Therapy* **1**, 3–8.

*Ellis, A. and Dryden, W. (1987) *The Practice of Rational-emotive Therapy*, New York: Springer.

Ellis, C. (1993) Incorporating the affective domain into staff development programs, *Journal of Nursing Staff Development* **9**(3), 127–30.

Ellis, R. and Whittington, D. (eds) (1983) *New Directions in Social Skills Training*, London: Croom Helm.

Emery, E. E. (1987) Empathy: psychoanalytic and client-centred, *American Psychologist* **42**, 513–15.

Erskine, R. and Moursund, J. (1988) *Integrative Psychotherapy in Action*, Newbury Park, CA: Sage Publications.

Evans, M. L. (1989) Simulations: their selection and use in developing nursing competencies, *Journal of Nursing Staff Development* **5**(2), 65–9.

Eysenck, H. J. (1992) The outcome problem in psychotherapy. In W. Dryden and C. Feltham (eds), *Psychotherapy and its Discontents*, Buckingham: Open University Press, 100–23.

Fagan, M. M. and Walter, G. (1982) Mentoring among teachers, *Journal of Educational Research* **76**(2), 113–18.

Farley, R. C. and Baker, A. J. (1987) Training on selected self-management techniques and the generalization and maintenance of interpersonal skills for registered nurse students, *Journal of Nursing Education* **26**(3), 104–7.

Firestone, R. W. (1988) A *Psychotherapeutic Approach to Self-destructive Behaviour*, New York: Human Sciences Press.

Fisch, R., Weakland, J. and Segal, L. (1985) *The Tactics of Change: Doing Therapy Briefly*, San Francisco: Jossey-Bass.

French, P. (1983) *Social Skills for Nursing Practice*, London: Croom Helm.

French, P. and Cross, D. (1992) An interpersonal epistemological curriculum model for nurse education, *Journal of Advanced Nursing* **17**(1), 83–9.

Gambrill, E (1984) Social skills training. In D. Larson (ed.), *Teaching Psychological Skills: Models for Giving Psychology Away*, Pacific Grove, CA: Brooks/Cole.

Gamel, C., Davis, B. and Hengeveld, M. (1993) Nurses' provision of teaching and counselling on sexuality: review of the literature, *Journal of Advanced Nursing* **18**(8), 1219–27.

Garfield, S. L. and Bergin, A. E. (1994) Introduction and historical overview. In A. E. Bergin and S. L. Garfield (eds), *Handbook of Psychotherapy and Behaviour Change*, 4th edn, Chichester: Wiley, 3–18.

Garvin, C. D. (1981) *Contemporary Group Work*, Englewood Cliffs, New Jersey: Prentice Hall.

Gaston, S. (1991) Sampling; an experiential learning activity, *Nurse Educator* **16**(5), 4, 12.

Gelatt, H. B. (1989) Positive uncertainty: a new decision-making framework for counselling, *Journal of Counselling Psychology* **36**, 252–6.

Gendlin, E. T. (1986) What comes after traditional psychotherapy research? *American Psychologist* **41**, 131–6.

George, P. and Kummerow, J. (1981) Mentoring for career women, *Training* **18**(2), 44–9.

Gibson, R. L. and Mitchell, M. H. (1986) *Introduction to Counselling and Guidance*, London: Collier Macmillan.

Gilbey, V. (1990) Screening and counselling clinic evaluation project, *Canadian Journal of Nursing Research* **22**(3), 23–38.

Gillam, T. (1993) Representational systems in counselling, *Nursing Standard* **8**(10), 25–7.

Goldfried, M. R., Greenberg, L. S. and Marmar, C. (1990) Individual psychotherapy: process and outcome, *Annual Review of Psychology* **41**, 659–88.

Gordon, D. (1982) The concept of the hidden curriculum, *Philosophy of Education* **16**(2), 187–8.

Gordon, S. and Waldo, M. (1984) The effects of assertive training on couples' relationships, *American Journal of Family Therapy* **12**, 73–7.

*Gould, D. (1990) Empathy: a review of the literature with suggestions for an alternative research strategy, *Journal of Advanced Nursing* **15**(10), 1167–74.

Greenberg, L. S. (1992) Task analysis: identifying components of interpersonal conflict resolution. In S. G. Toukmanian and D. L. Rennie (eds), *Psychotherapy Process Research: Paradigmatic and Narrative Approaches*, London: Sage, 22–50.

Greenberg, L. S. and Pinsof, W. M. (eds) (1986) *The Psychotherapeutic Process: A Research Handbook*, New York: Guilford Press.

Greenwood, J. (1993a) Reflective practice: a critique of the work of Argyris and Schon, *Journal of Advanced Nursing*, **18**(8), 1183–7.

Greenwood, J. (1993b) Some considerations concerning practice and feedback in nursing education, *Journal of Advanced Nursing* **18**(12), 1999–2000.

Grencavage, L. N. and Norcross, J. C. (1990) Where are the commonalities among the therapeutic common factors?, *Professional Psychology: Research and Practice* **21**, 372–8.

Guccione, A. A. and DeMont, M. E. (1987) Interpersonal skills education in entry-level physical therapy programs, *Physical Therapy* **67**(3), 388–93.

Guinn, C. A. (1992) Experiential learning: a 'real-world' introduction for baccalaureate nursing students, *Nurse Educator* **17**(3), 31, 36.

Hardin, S. I., Subich, L. M. and Holvey, J. M. (1988) Expectancies for counselling in relation to premature termination, *Journal of Counselling Psychology* **35**, 37–40.

Hare, A. P. (1976) *Handbook of Small Group Research*, New York: Free Press.

*Hargie, O. (ed.) (1986) *A Handbook of Communication Skills*, London: Croom Helm.

Henry, W. P., Strupp, H. H., Schact, T. E. and Gaston, L. (1994) Psychodynamic approaches. In A. E. Bergin and S. L. Garfield (eds), *Handbook of Psychotherapy and Behaviour Change*, 4th edn, New York: Wiley, 467–508.

Heppner, P. P. (1989) Identifying the complexities within clients' thinking and decision making, *Journal of Counselling Psychology* **36**, 257–9.

Heppner, P. P. and Krauskopf, C. J. (1987) An information-processing approach to personal problem solving. *Counselling Psychologist* **15**, 371–447.

Heppner, P. P., Kivlighan Jr, D.M. and Wampold, B. E. (1992) *Research Design in Counselling*, Pacific Grove, CA: Brooks/Cole.

Hill, C. E. (1989) *Therapist Techniques and Client Outcomes: Eight Cases of Brief Psychotherapy*, London: Sage.

Hill, C. E. (1991) Almost everything you ever wanted to know about how to do process research on counselling and psychotherapy but didn't know who to ask. In C. E. Watkins and L. J. Schneider (eds) *Research in Counselling*, Hillsdale, NJ: Lawrence Erlbaum, 85–118.

Hill C. E. and Corbett, M. M. (1993) A perspective on the history of process and outcome research in counselling psychology, *Journal of Counselling Psychology* **32**, 3–22.

Holt, R. (1982) An alternative to mentorship, *Adult Education* **55**(2), 152–6.

Hopper, E. (1991) Shattered dreams ... counselling work with bereaved parents, *Nursing Standard* **6**(4), 20–1.

Houle, C. O. (1984) *Patterns of Learning*, San Francisco: Jossey Bass.

Hunt, P. (1985) *Clients' Responses to Marriage Counselling*, Rugby: NMGC.

Ivey, A. E. (1987) *Counselling and Psychotherapy: Skills, Theories and Practice*, London: Prentice Hall International.

Jacob, M. R. (1988) Putting research into practice: the impact of interpersonal skills training on responses to patients' emotional concerns by nursing staff in a general hospital, *Florida Nurse* **36**(9), 18.

Jacobson, N. S., Follette, W. C. and Revenstorf, D. (1984) Psychotherapy outcome research: methods for reporting variability and evaluating clinical significance, *Behaviour Therapy* **15**, 336—52.

Jarvis, P. (1983a) *Professional Education*, London: Croom Helm.

Jarvis, P. (1983b) *The Theory and Practice of Adult and Continuing Education*, London: Croom Helm.

*Jarvis, P. (1985) *The Sociology of Adult and Continuing Education*, London: Croom Helm.

Jarvis, P. (1987) Meaningful and meaningless experience: towards an understanding of learning from life, *Adult Education Quarterly* **37**(3).

Jeavons, B. (1991) Developing counselling skills, *Nursing (London), The Journal of Clinical Practice Education and Management* **4**(38), 28–9.

Jenkins, D. and Shipman, M. D. (1976) *Curriculum: An Introduction*, London: Open Books.

Johns, C. (1993a) On becoming effective in taking ethical action, *Journal of Clinical Nursing* **2**(5), 307–12.

Johns, C. (1993b) Professional supervision, *Journal of Nursing Management* **1**(1), 9–18.

Johnson, D. W. and Johnson, F. P. (1982) *Joining Together*, 2nd edn, Englewood Cliffs, New Jersey: Prentice Hall.

Jones, A. (1991) The path towards a common goal: structuring the counselling process, *Professional Nurse* **6**(6), 302, 304–6.

Jones, A. (1992) Confronting the inevitable ... counselling ... a patient, *Nursing Standard* **6**(46), 54–6.

Jones, A. (1993) A first step in effective communication: providing a supportive environment for counselling in hospital, *Professional Nurse* **8**(8), 501–2, 502–5.

Jones, C. (1990) All you ever wanted to know about ... counselling, *Nursing Times*, 55–8.

Jones, J. (1991) Therapeutic use of metaphor, *Nursing Standard*, **6**(11), 30–2.

Kagan, N. (1984) Interpersonal process recall: basic methods and recent research. In D. Larsen (ed.), *Teaching Psychological Skills*, Monterey, CA: Brooks/Cole.

Kanfer, F. H. and Schefft, B. K. (1988) *Guiding Therapeutic Change*, Champaign, IL: Research Press.

Kazdin, A. E. (1994) Methodology, design and evaluation in psychotherapy research. In A. E. Bergin and S. L. Garfield (eds), *Handbook of Psychotherapy and Behaviour Change*, 4th edn, Chichester: Wiley, 19–71.

Kendall, P. C. and Hollon, S. D. (eds) (1981) *Assessment Strategies for Cognitive Behavioural Interventions*, New York: Academic Press.

Kilty, J. (1987) *Staff Development for Nurse Education: Practitioners Supporting Staff*, Human Potential Research Project, Guildford: University of Surrey.

Klopf, G. J. and Harrison, J. (1981) Moving up the career ladder: the case for mentors, *Principal* **61**(1), 41–3.

Knight, J. (1992) The lecturer practitioner [sic] role: exploration and reflection, *Journal of Clinical Nursing*, **1**(2), 58–9.

Knox, A. B. (ed.) (1980) *Teaching Adults Effectively*, San Francisco, California: Jossey Bass.

Kottler, J. A. (1986) *On Being a Therapist*, San Francisco: Jossey-Bass.

Kramer, M. K. (1993) Concept clarification and critical thinking: integrated processes, *Journal of Nursing Education* **32**(9), 406–14.

Kutash, I. L. and Wolf, A. (eds) (1986) *The Psychotherapist's Casbook*, San Francisco: Jossey-Bass.

L'Abate, L. and Milan, M. (eds) (1985) *Handbook of Social Skills Training and Research*, New York: Wiley.

Lambert, M. J., Masters, K. S. and Ogles, B. M. (1991) Outcome research in counselling. In C. E. Watkins and L. J. Schneider (eds), *Research in Counselling*, Hillsdale, NJ: Lawrence Erlbaum, 51–84.

Larson, V. A. (1987) An exploration of psychotherapeutic resonance, *Psychotherapy* **24**, 321–4.

Legge, D. (1982) *The Education of Adults in Britain*, Milton Keynes: Open University Press.

Levine, A. (1985) The Pollyana paradigm, *Journal of Humanistic Psychology* **25**(1), 90–3.

Liberman, R. P., King, L. W., DeRisi, W. J. and McCann, M. (1976) *Personal Effectiveness*, Champagne: Research Press.

Lietaer, G. (1991) Client-centred/experiential psychotherapy and counselling bibliographic survey 1988–90, *Psychotherapeutische Bijdragen*, Report No. 6.

Lietaer, G. (1992) Helping and hindering processes in client-centred/experiential psychotherapy: a content analysis of client and therapist postsession perceptions. In S. G. Toukmanian and D. L. Rennie (eds) *Psychotherapy Process Research: Paradigmatic and Narrative Approaches*, London: Sage, 134–62.

Lindsey, E. and Attridge, C. (1989) Staff nurses' perceptions of support in an acute care workplace, *Canadian Journal of Nursing Research* **21**(2), 15–25.

Lister, P. (1989) Experiential learning and the benefits of journal work, *Senior Nurse* **9**(6), 20–1.

Lopez, K. A. (1983) Role modelling interpersonal skills with beginning nursing students: Gestalt techniques, *Journal of Nursing Education* **22**(3), 119–22.

Luborsky, L. (1984) *Principles of Psychotherapy: A Manual for Supportive-Expressive Treatment*, New York: Basic Books.

Luborsky, L. (1993) Recommendations for training therapists based on manuals for psychotherapy research, *Psychotherapy* **30**(4), 578—80.

Luborsky, L. and DeRubeis, R. J. (1984) The use of psychotherapy treatment manuals: a small revolution in psychotherapy research style, *Clinical Psychology Review* 54f, 39–47.

Macaskill, N. and Macaskill, A. (1992) Psychotherapists-in-training evaluate their personal therapy: results of a UK survey, *British Journal of Psychotherapy* **9**(2), 133–8.

McCamiele, R. (ed.) (1982) *Calling Education into Account*, London: Heinemann.

McCaugherty, D. (1991) The use of a teaching model to promote reflection and the experiential integration of theory and practice in first-year student-nurses: an action research study, *Journal of Advanced Nursing* **16**(5), 534–43.

McGregor, D. (1960) *The Human Side of Enterprise*, New York: McGraw-Hill.

McGuire, J. and Priestley, P. (1981) *Life After School: A Social Skills Curriculum*, Oxford: Pergamon.

McIntosh, A. (1982) Psychology and adult education. In S. Canter and D. Canter (eds), *Psychology in Practice*, Chichester: Wiley.

McLeod, J. (1992) The story of Henry Murray's diagnostic council: a case study in the demise of a scientific method, *Clinical Psychology Forum* **44** (June), 6–12.

*McLeod, J. (1994a) The research agenda for counselling, *Counselling* **5**(1), 41–3.

McLeod, J. (1994b) Issues in the organisation of counselling: learning from NMGC, *British Journal of Guidance and Counselling* **22**(2), 163–74.

McMillan, I. (1991) A listening ear ... telephone counselling, *Nursing Times* **87**(6), 30–1.

McWilliams, S. (1991) Affective changes following severe head injury as perceived by patients and relatives, *British Journal of Occupational Therapy* **54**(7), 246–8.

Maguire, P. (1991) Managing difficult communication tasks. In R. Corney (ed.), *Developing Communication Skills in Medicine*, London: Routledge.

*Mahrer, A. and Nadler, W. (1986) Good moments in psychotherapy: a preliminary review, a list and some promising research avenues, *Journal of Consulting and Clinical Psychology* **54**(1), 10–5.

Mander, R. (1992) See how they learn: experience as the basis of practice, *Nurse Education Today* **121**, 3–10.

Marks, S. E. and Tolsma, R. J. (1986) Empathy research: some methodological considerations, *Psychotherapy* **23**, 4–20.

Marshall, E. K. and Kurtz, P. D. (eds) (1982) *Interpersonal Helping Skills: A Guide to Training Methods, Programs and Resources*, San Francisco, California: Jossey Bass.

Marte, A. L. (1991) Experiential Learning strategies for promoting positive staff attitudes toward the elderly, *Journal of Continuing Education in Nursing* **22**(2), 73–7.

Martin, J., Martin, W. and Slemon, A. G. (1989) Cognitive-mediational models of action-act sequences in counselling, *Journal of Counselling Psychology* **36**, 8–16.

Marziali, E. A. (1987) People in your life: development of a social support measure for predicting psychotherapy outcome, *Journal of Nervous and Mental Disease* **175**, 313–26.

Meara, N. M. and Thorne, B. (1988) *Person-Centred Counselling in Action*, London: Sage.

Melby, V. (1992) Counselling of patients with HIV related diseases: what if the role of the nurse?, *Journal of Clinical Nursing* **1**(1), 39–45.

Merriam, S. (1984) Mentors and protégés: a critical review of the literature, *Adult Education Quarterly* **33**(3), 161–73.

Mezeiro, J. (1981) A critical theory of adult learning and education, *Adult Education* **32**(1), 3–24.

Millar, R., Goldman, E., Bor, R. and Scher, I. (1992) Counselling in terminal care, *Nursing Standard* **6**(26), AIDS Focus, 52–5.

Miller, R. (1993) Bereavement counselling in HIV disease, *Nursing Standard* **7**(39), AIDS Focus, 48–51.

Morsund, J. (1985) *The Process of Counselling and Therapy*, Englewood Cliffs, New Jersey: Prentice Hall.

*Murgatroyd, S. (1986) *Counselling and Helping*, London: British Psychological Society and Methuen.

*Murgatroyd, S. and Woolfe, R. (1982) *Coping with Crisis – Understanding and Helping Persons in Need*, London: Harper & Row.

*Myerscough, P. R. (1989) *Talking with Patients: A Basic Clinical Skill*, Oxford: Oxford Medical Publications.

Nadler, L. (ed.) (1984) *The Handbook of Human Resource Development*, New York: Wiley.

Newell, R. and Dryden, W. (1991) Clinical problems: an introduction to the cognitive-behavioural approach. In W. Dryden and R. Rentoul (eds), *Clinical Problems: A Cognitive-behavioural Approach*, London: Routledge.

Newell, R. (1992) Anxiety, accuracy and reflection: the limits of professional development, *Journal of Advanced Nursing* **17**(11), 1326–33.

*Newell, R. (1994) *Interviewing Skills for Nurses and Other Health Care Professionals: A Structured Approach*, London: Routledge.

Nkowane, A. M. (1993) Breaking the silence: the need for counselling of HIV/AIDS patients, *International Nursing Review* **40**(1), 17–20, 24.

Nyatanga, L. (1989) Experiential taxonomy and experiential learning, *Senior Nurse* **9**(8), 24–7.

Nytanga, L. (1989) Social skills training: some ideas on its origin, nature and application, *Nurse Education Today* **9**(1), 56–63.

Ohlsen, A. M., Horne, A. M. and Lawe, C. F. (1988) *Group Counselling*, New York: Holt Rinehart & Winston.

Olson, J. K. and Iwasiw, C. L. (1987) Effects of a training model on active listening skills of post-RN students, *Journal of Nursing Education* **26**(3), 104–7.

Omer, H. and Dar, R. (1992) Changing trends in three decades of psychotherapy research: the flight from theory into pragmatics, *Journal of Consulting and Clinical Psychology* **60**, 88–93.

*Open University Coping With Crisis Group (1987) *Running Workshops: A Guide for Trainers in the Helping Professions*, London: Croom Helm.

Orlinsky, D. E. (1989) Researchers' images of psychotherapy: their origins and influence on research, *Clinical Psychology Review* **9**, 413–41.

Osborn, T. (1984) The question of peer assessment: self and society, *European Journal of Humanistic Psychology* **12**(4), 201–6.

Palmer, M. E. and Deck, E. S. (1982) Assertiveness education: one method for teaching staff and patients, *Nurse Educator*, Winter, 36–9.

Parry, G. (1992) Improving psychotherapy services: applications of research, audit and evaluation, *British Journal of Clinical Psychology* **31**, 3–19.

Patterson, C. H. (1984) Empathy, warmth and genuineness in psychotherapy: a review of reviews, *Psychotherapy* **21**, 431–8.

Patton, M. Q. (1982) *Practical Evaluation*, Beverly Hills, California: Sage.

Paunonen, M. (1991) Testing a model for counsellor training in three public health care organisations, *Nurse Education Today* **11**(4), 270–7.

Pearson, R. E. (1983) Support groups: a conceptualization, *Personnel and Guidance Journal* **61**, 361–4.

Pekarik, G. and Wierzbicki, M. (1986) The relationship between clients' expected and actual treatment duration, *Psychotherapy* **23**, 532–4.

Philips, K. and Fraser, T. (1982) *The Management of Interpersonal Skills Training*, Aldershot: Gower.

Phillip-Jones, L. (1982) *Mentors and Protégés*, New York: Arbor House.

Phillip-Jones, L. (1983) Establishing a formalised mentoring programme, *Training and Development Journal*, Feb., 38–42.

Phillips, J. (1993) Counselling and the nurse, *British Journal of Theatre Nursing* **2**(10), **13**(4).

Pope, B. (1986) *Social Skills Training for Psychiatric Nurses*, London: Harper & Row.

Priestley, P., McQuire, J., Flegg, D., Hemsley, V. and Welham, D. (1978) *Social Skills and Personal Problem Solving*, London: Tavistock.

Pulsford, D. (1993a) Reducing the threat: an experiential exercise to introduce role play to student nurses, *Nurse Education Today* **13**(2), 145–8.

Pulsford, D. (1993b) The reluctant participant in experiential learning, *Nurse Education Today* **13**(2), 139–44.

Ramos, M. C. (1992) The nurse-patient relationship: theme and variations, *Journal of Advanced Nursing* **17**, 496–506.

Rawlings, M. E. and Rawlings, L. (1983) Mentoring and networking for helping professionals, *Personnel and Guidance Journal* **62**(2), 116–18.

Reddy, M. (1987) *The Manager's Guide to Counselling at Work*, London: Methuen.

Rennie, D. L. (1994a) Clients' deference in psychotherapy, *Journal of Counselling Psychology*, in press.

Rennie, D. L. (1994b) Storytelling in psychotherapy: the client's subjective experience, *Psychotherapy* **31**, 234–43.

Richards, D. A. and McDonald, R. (1990) *Behavioural Psychotherapy: A Handbook for Nurses*, Oxford: Heinemann.

Ricketts, T. (1993) Therapist self-disclosure in behavioural psychotherapy, *British Journal of Nursing*, **2**(13), 667–71.

Robotham, A. (1992) The use of credit and experiential learning in nurse education: exciting opportunities for student and tutor alike, *Nurse Education Today*, **11**(6), 448–53.

Rogers, J. C. (1982) Sponsorship – developing leaders for occupational therapy, *American Journal of Occupational Therapy* **36**, 309–13.

Rolfe, G. (1990a) The assessment of therapeutic attitudes in the psychiatric setting, *Journal of Advanced Nursing* **15**(5), 564–70.

Rolfe, G. (1990b) The role of clinical supervision in the education of student psychiatric nurses: a theoretical approach, *Nurse Education Today* **10**(3), 193–7.

Rusk, T. and Rusk, N. (1988) *Mind Traps: Change Your Mind, Change Your Life*, Los Angeles: Price, Stern & Sloan.

Russell, R. L. (1989) Language and psychotherapy, *Clinical Psychology Review* **9**, 505–20.

Sampson Jr, J. P. (1991) The place of the computer in counselling research. In C. E. Watkins and L. J. Schneider (eds), *Research in Counselling*, Hilldfslr, NJ: Lawrence Erlbaum, 261–86.

Satow, A. and Evans, M. (1983) *Working with Groups*, Manchester: Tacade.

Schmidt, J. A. and Wolfe, J. S. (1980) The mentor partnership: discovery of professionalism, *NASPA Journal* **17**, 45–51.

Schon, D. A. (1987) *Educating the Reflective Practitioner: Towards a New Design for Teaching and Learning in the Professions*, San Francisco: Jossey-Bass.

Shamian, J. and Inhaber, R. (1985) The concept and practice of preceptorship in contemporary nursing: a review of pertinent literature, *The International Journal of Nursing Studies* **22**(2), 79–88.

Shapiro, S. B. (1985) An empirical analysis of operating values in humanistic education, *Journal of Humanistic Psychology* **25**(1), 94–108.

Shaw, M. E. (1981) *Group Dynamics: The Psychology of Small Group Behaviour*, New York: McGraw-Hill.

Shoham-Salomon, V. and Rosenthal, R. (1987) Paradoxical interventions: a meta-analysis, *Journal of Consulting and Clinical Psychology*, **55**, 22–8.

Shropshire, C. O. (1981) Group experiential learning in adult education, *The Journal of Continuing Education in Nursing* **12**(6), 5–9.

Skovholt, T. M. and Ronnestad, M. H. (1992) *The Evolving Professional Self: Stages and Themes in Therapist and Counselor Development*, New York: Wiley.

Sloboda, J. A., Hopkins, J. S., Turner, A., Rogers, D. and McLeod, J. (1993) An evaluated staff counselling programme in a public sector organisation, *Employee Counselling Today* **5**(5), 4–12.

Smith, P. B. (1980) *Group Processes and Personal Change*, Harper & Row, London.

Snyder, M. (1993) Critical thinking: a foundation for consumer-focused care, *Journal of Continuing Education in Nursing*, **24**(5), 206–10.

Speck, P. (1992) Managing the boundaries...using our counselling skills to help a colleague or a student can create more problems, *Nursing Times* **88**(32), 22.

Speizer, J. J. (1981) Role models, mentors and sponsors: the elusive concept, *Signs* **6**, 692–712.

Steenbarger, B. N. (1992) Toward science-practice integration in brief counselling and psychotherapy, *Counselling Psychologist* **20**, 403–50.

Stiles, W. B., Elliott, R., Llewellyn, S., Firth-Cozens, J., Margison, F., Shapiro, D. A. and Hardy, G. (1990) Assimilation of problematic experiences by clients in psychotherapy, *Psychotherapy* **27**, 411–20.

Stitch, T. F. (1983) Experiential therapy, *Journal of Experiential Education*, **5**(3), 23–30.

Sweeney, J. A., Clarkin, J. F. and Fitzgibbon, M. L. (1987) Current practice of psychological assessment, *Professional Psychology, Research and Practice* **18**, 377–80.

Taylor, S. (1986) Mentors: who are they and what are they doing?, *Thrust For Educational Leadership* **15**(7), 39–41.

Thomas, E. J. (1984) *Designing Interventions for the Helping Professions*, Beverly Hills: Sage.

Thorne, B. and Dryden, W. (eds) (1993) *Counselling: Interdisciplinary Perspectives*, Buckingham: Open University Press.

Thorne, P. (1991) Assessment of prior experiential learning, *Nursing Standard* **6**(10), 32–4.

Timms, N. and Blampied, A. (1985) *Intervention in Marriage: The Experience of Counsellors and their Clients*, University of Sheffield: Joint Unit for Social Services Research.

Toukmanian, S. G. (1992) Studying the client's perceptual processes and their outcomes in psychotherapy. In S. G. Toukmanian and D. L. Rennie (eds), *Psychotherapy Process Research: Paradigmatic and Narrative Approaches*, London: Sage, 77–107.

Trower, P., O'Mahony, J. M. and Dryden, W. (1982) Cognitive aspects of social failure: some implications for social skills training, *British Journal of Guidance and Counselling* **10**, 176–84.

Truax, C. B. and Carkhuff, R. R. (1967) *Toward Effective Counselling and Psychotherapy: Training and Practice*, Chicago: Aldine.

*Van Deurzen-Smith, E. (1988) *Existential counselling in practice*, Newbury Park, CA: Sage Publications.

Vandecreek, L. and Angstadt, L. (1985) Client preferences and anticipations about counselor self-disclosure, *Journal of Counselling Psychology* **32**, 206–14.

Vauderslott, J. (1992) A supportive therapy that undermines violence: counselling to prevent ward violence, *Professional Nurse*, **7**(7), 427–8, 430.

Victor, C. *et al.* (1993) Improving counselling skills: training in obstetric and paediatric HIV and AIDS, *Professional Care of Mother and Child* **3**(4), 97–100.

Victor, C., Jefferies, S. and Sherr, L. (1993) Improving counselling skills: training in obstetric and paediatric HIV and AIDS, *Professional Care of Mother and Child*, **3**(4), 97–100.

Ward, D. E. (1984) Termination of individual counselling: concepts and strategies, *Journal of Counselling and Development* **63**, 21–5.

Weinstein, G. and Alschuler, A. S. (1985) Educating and counselling for self-knowledge development, *Journal of Counselling and Development* **64**, 19–25.

Wilkins, H. (1993) Transcultural nursing: a selective review of the literature: 1985–1991, *Journal of Advanced Nursing* **184**, 602–12.

Wilkinson, J. and Canter, S. (1982) *Social Skills Training Manual: Assessment, Programme Design and Management of Training*, Wiley: Chichester.

Wlodkowski, R. J. (1985) *Enhancing Adult Motivation to Learn*, San Francisco, California: Jossey Bass.

Wondrak, R. and Goble, J. (1992) An investigation into self, peer and tutor assessments of student psychiatric nurses written work assignments, *Nurse Education Today* **12**(1), 61–4.

Wright, J. (1991) Counselling at the cultural interface: is getting back to roots enough?, *Journal of Advanced Nursing* 16(1), 92–100.

Wyatt, P. (1993) The role of nurses in counselling the terminally ill patient, *British Journal of Nursing* **2**(14), 701–4.

Zander, A. (1982) *Making Groups Effective*, San Francisco: Jossey Bass.

Index